*Study Guide to Accompany*

# Foundations
# of Basic Nursing
## Third Edition

*Study Guide to Accompany*

# Foundations of Basic Nursing

## Third Edition

### Lois White, RN, PhD,

### Gena Duncan, MSEd, MSN,

### Wendy Baumle, MSN

**Prepared by**
**Cheryl Pratt, RN, MA, CNAA-BC**
**Regional Director of Nursing**
**School of Nursing**
**Rasmussen College**

**Previous edition prepared by**
**Kathleen Peck Schaefer, RNC, MSN, MEd**
**Brandy Coward, BSN**

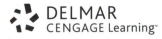

DELMAR
CENGAGE Learning™

Australia • Brazil • Japan • Korea • Mexico • Singapore • Spain • United Kingdom • United States

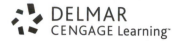

**Foundations of Basic Nursing Study Guide, Third Edition**

**By Lois White, RN, PhD, Gena Duncan, MSEd, MSN, and Wendy Baumle, MSN**

Vice President, Career and Professional Editorial: Dave Garza

Director of Learning Solutions: Matt Kane

Executive Editor: Steven Helba

Managing Editor: Marah Bellegarde

Senior Product Manager: Juliet Steiner

Editorial Assistant: Meghan E. Orvis

Vice President, Career and Professional Marketing: Jennifer Ann Baker

Executive Marketing Manager: Wendy Mapstone

Senior Marketing Manager: Michele McTighe

Marketing Coordinator: Scott Chrysler

Production Director: Carolyn Miller

Production Manager: Andrew Crouth

Senior Content Project Manager: James Zayicek

Senior Art Director: Jack Pendleton

For product information and technology assistance, contact us at **Professional & Career Group Customer Support, 1-800-648-7450**

For permission to use material from this text or product, submit all requests online at **cengage.com/permissions**. Further permissions questions can be e-mailed to **permissionrequest@cengage.com**.

Library of Congress Control Number: 2009929886
ISBN-13: 978-1-4283-1783-3
ISBN-10: 1-4283-1783-X

**Delmar**
5 Maxwell Drive
Clifton Park, NY 12065-2919
USA

Cengage Learning products are represented in Canada by Nelson Education, Ltd.

For your lifelong learning solutions, visit **delmar.cengage.com**
Visit our corporate website at **cengage.com**.

**NOTICE TO THE READER**

Publisher does not warrant or guarantee any of the products described herein or perform any independent analysis in connection with any of the product information contained herein. Publisher does not assume, and expressly disclaims, any obligation to obtain and include information other than that provided to it by the manufacturer. The reader is expressly warned to consider and adopt all safety precautions that might be indicated by the activities described herein and to avoid all potential hazards. By following the instructions contained herein, the reader willingly assumes all risks in connection with such instructions. The publisher makes no representations or warranties of any kind, including but not limited to, the warranties of fitness for particular purpose or merchantability, nor are any such representations implied with respect to the material set forth herein, and the publisher takes no responsibility with respect to such material. The publisher shall not be liable for any special, consequential, or exemplary damages resulting, in whole or part, from the readers' use of, or reliance upon, this material.

Printed in the United States of America
1 2 3 4 5 6 7 14 13 12 11 10

# Contents

# Preface

This Study Guide is designed to accompany *Foundations of Basic Nursing*, Third Edition, by Lois White, Gena Duncan, and Wendy Baumle. Each of the 31 chapters in this guide was created to facilitate student learning and refine student skills. By using this guide at home and in the clinical setting, you will work with important concepts and begin to apply them to real-life situations.

To facilitate your learning, each chapter in this guide includes the following components:

- *Key Terms Review*: a matching exercise designed to enhance your understanding of new terms presented in the text.
- *Abbreviation Review*: exercise to test your knowlege of abbreviations, acronyms, and symbols used in the text.
- *Exercises and Activities*: short scenarios with related questions to test your understanding and application of concepts.
- *Self-Assessment Questions*: multiple-choice questions that draw on the key ideas in the chapter and prepare you to succeed in your examinations.

# Student Nurse Skills for Success

## Key Terms

Match the following terms with their correct definitions.

___ 1. Ability

___ 2. Accountability

___ 3. Anxiety

___ 4. Assignment

___ 5. Attitude

___ 6. Attribute

___ 7. Critical thinking

___ 8. Delegation

___ 9. Disciplined

___10. Encoding

___11. Judgment

___12. Learning

___12. Learning disability

___14. Learning style

___15. Mnemonic

___16. Opinion

a. System to help meet goals through problem solving.

b. Method to aid in association and recall; a memorable sentence created from the first letters of a list of items to be used to recall the items later.

c. Act or process of acquiring knowledge and/or skill in a particular subject.

d. Physiological response of the autonomic nervous system to a perceived stressful situation.

e. A level or degree of quality.

f. Intentionally putting off or delaying something that should be done.

g. Subjective beliefs.

h. Characteristic that belongs to an individual.

i. Heterogeneous group of disorders manifested by significant difficulties in the acquisition and use of listening, speaking, reading, writing, reasoning, or mathematical abilities.

j. The disciplined intellectual process of applying skillful reasoning, imposing intellectual standards, and using self-reflective thinking as a guide to a belief or an action.

k. Overwhelming expectation of being able to get everything done.

l. Individual preference for receiving, processing, and assimilating information about a particular subject.

m. Laying down tracks in areas of the brain to enhance the ability to recall and utilize information.

n. Manner, feeling, or position toward a person or thing.

o. Competence in an activity.

p. Conclusions based on sound reasoning and supported by evidence.

___17. Perfectionism

___18. Procrastination

___19. Reasoning

___20. Standards

___21. Time management

q. Trained by instruction and exercise.

r. Use of the elements of thought to solve a problem or settle a question.

s. Responsibility for actions and inactions performed by oneself or others.

t. The transfer of activities from one person to another.

u. Process of tranferring a select nursing task to a licensed individual who is competent to perform that specified task.

## Abbreviation Review

Write the meaning or definition of the following abbreviations/acronyms.

1. BP _____

2. CAI _____

3. NCLEX-PN _____

4. ATT _____

5. UAP _____

6. NCSBN _____

7. CNA _____

## Exercises and Activities

1. In the first column, list the abilities and skills you believe are useful or necessary to be a competent nurse. In the second column, list the abilities and skills you will need to be a successful student.

_Nurse_                                         _Student_

2. Using the list of skills in the first column, write at least three examples of how each skill might be used in nursing in the second column (skills may be combined in an example).

| _Skills_ | _Examples in Nursing_ |
| --- | --- |
| Reading | |
| Mathematics | |
| Writing | |
| Listening | |
| Speaking | |

3. Rewrite each of these negative statements into positive ones that encourage problem solving and goal-oriented behavior.

   a. "I can't understand math equations."

   _____

   b. "I have too much homework to do."

   _____

   c. "I can't stay awake in that class."

   _____

   d. "I don't understand what the teacher is saying."

   _____

   e. "The teacher goes through the material too fast."

   _____

   f. "I'm never going to be able to learn all of this."

   _____

   g. "I know I'm going to do poorly on this exam."

   _____

4. Reread the descriptions of the two classroom settings in your core text in the section entitled "Develop Your Learning Style." Professor A uses a variety of teaching techniques, and Professor B relies on a straight lecture format. Now imagine that you are a student in Professor B's class. List several strategies that you could use to enhance your learning in this class. Include ideas that relate to different learning styles.

   _____

   _____

   _____

   _____

5. Use the following time graph and personalize it for your class and clinical schedule. Don't forget to include class time, lecture and clinical work, religious activities, family commitments, study time, and transportation.

|        | *Sunday* | *Monday* | *Tuesday* | *Wednesday* | *Thursday* | *Friday* | *Saturday* |
|--------|----------|----------|-----------|-------------|------------|----------|------------|
| 7 A.M. |          |          |           |             |            |          |            |
| 8 A.M. |          |          |           |             |            |          |            |
| 9 A.M. |          |          |           |             |            |          |            |
| 10 A.M.|          |          |           |             |            |          |            |

*continued*

| | Sunday | Monday | Tuesday | Wednesday | Thursday | Friday | Saturday |
|---|---|---|---|---|---|---|---|
| 11 A.M. | | | | | | | |
| 12 P.M. | | | | | | | |
| 1 P.M. | | | | | | | |
| 2 P.M. | | | | | | | |
| 3 P.M. | | | | | | | |
| 4 P.M. | | | | | | | |
| 5 P.M. | | | | | | | |
| 6 P.M. | | | | | | | |
| 7 P.M. | | | | | | | |
| 8 P.M. | | | | | | | |
| 9 P.M. | | | | | | | |
| 10 P.M. | | | | | | | |
| 11 P.M. | | | | | | | |

What is your best study time? _____ Is that reflected in your schedule?

List three of your own personal time wasters and a strategy for each that could help you reclaim some of that time.

| | **Time Waster** | **Strategy** |
|---|---|---|
| (1) | | |
| (2) | | |
| (3) | | |

List two activities that you could delegate to others.

(1) _____

(2) _____

6. As a new (licensed practical/vocational nurse), you are caring for your client, Mrs. Thompson, a new mother who delivered her first baby yesterday evening. You note that Mrs. Thompson appears to be somewhat tired this morning, but very excited about her new baby. Although somewhat nervous about caring for her new baby, she asks you to show her how to give her baby a bath. The baby is awake but quiet—this is the perfect time. What teaching strategy could you include for each of the following learning styles to help Mrs. Thompson learn how to bathe her baby?

Visual: _____

_____

Auditory: _____

_____

Kinesthetic: _____

_____

7. The process of critical thinking is based on developing the following four skills: critical reading, critical listening, critical writing, and critical speaking.

   a. List two tactics that will help you to develop critical reading skills.

      (1) _____

      (2) _____

   b. Write two suggestions to improve your critical listening skills.

      (1) _____

      (2) _____

   c. List two critical thinking standards that evaluate the quality of your critical writing technique.

      (1) _____

      (2) _____

   d. Give two actions that should be avoided in critical speaking.

      (1) _____

      (2) _____

## Self-Assessment Questions

Circle the letter that corresponds to the best answer.

1. Mild anxiety may cause a student to
   a. be more easily distracted.
   b. focus on small or scattered details.
   c. feel alert and motivated.
   d. lose a sense of the "whole."

2. It is crucial for a student who may have a learning disability to
   a. focus on application of information.
   b. develop alternative learning styles.
   c. become a kinesthetic learner.
   d. get professional testing.

3. Being able to summarize a writer's message shows evidence of
   a. basic competency.
   b. accuracy.
   c. comprehension.
   d. metacognition.

4. A student who has practiced testing skills for the NCLEX-PN will
   a. attempt to identify priorities correctly.
   b. infer additional data from experiences.
   c. first scan questions to determine difficulty level.
   d. establish agreement or disagreement with the question.

5. A nurse caring for several ill patients with multiple needs may rely primarily on
   a. skill building.
   b. time management skills.
   c. help from colleagues.
   d. goal setting.

6. A student who is learning to give an injection demonstrates a kinesthetic learning strategy by
   a. studying injection techniques with a small group of students.
   b. watching a nurse give an injection to a client.
   c. demonstrating an injection on a laboratory mannequin.
   d. developing a chart on various types of injection techniques.

7. Select the strategy not suited to getting the most from class.
   a. Write definitions and mathematical formulas exactly as you heard them.
   b. Pick an abbreviation system and stick to it.
   c. Condense the amount of actual writing.
   d. Take notes with the intent of writing them over.

8. Which of the following is *not* a trait of a disciplined thinker?
   a. Courage
   b. Sympathy
   c. Integrity
   d. Perseverance

9. Which of the five rights of delegation deals with the availability of resources?
   a. Right task
   b. Right circumstance
   c. Right person
   d. Right direction/communication
   e. Right supervision

10. Who cannot perform a task that falls within the protected scope of practice of any licensed profession?
    a. RN
    b. NP
    c. VN
    d. UAP

# Holistic Care

## Key Terms

Match the following terms with their correct definitions.

____ 1. Attitude

____ 2. Body mechanics

____ 3. Culture

____ 4. Health

____ 5. Health continuum

____ 6. Holistic

____ 7. Homeostasis

____ 8. Intellectual wellness

____ 9. Maslow's Hierarchy of Needs

____10. Physical wellness

____11. Psychological wellness

____12. Self-awareness

____13. Self-concept

____14. Sociocultural wellness

____15. Spiritual wellness

____16. Wellness

a. Inner strength and peace.

b. Enjoyment of creativity, satisfaction of the basic need to love and be loved, understanding of emotions, and ability to maintain control over emotions.

c. Whole; includes physical, intellectual, sociocultural, psychological, and spiritual aspects as an integrated whole.

d. Theory of behavioral motivation based on needs; includes physiological, safety and security, love and belonging, self-esteem, and self-actualization needs.

e. A feeling about people, places, or things that is evident in the way one behaves.

f. Consciously knowing how the self thinks, feels, believes, and behaves at any specific time.

g. Balance or stability that the body strives to achieve with mind and spirit.

h. Behavior, customs, and beliefs of the family, extended family, tribe, nation, and society.

i. Use of the body to move or lift objects.

j. How a person thinks or feels about himself.

k. A healthy body that functions at an optimal level.

l. Ability to function as an independent person capable of making sound decisions.

m. State of an organism performing its vital functions normally and properly.

n. Ability to appreciate the needs of others and to care about one's environment and the inhabitants of it.

o. Highest potential for personal health.

p. Range of an individual's health, from highest health potential to death.

## Abbreviation Review

Write the meaning or definition of the following abbreviations.

1. AHNA _____

2. CDC _____

3. NIH _____

4. OAM _____

5. WHO _____

6. NCCAM _____

## Exercises and Activities

1. Describe the term *holistic health.*

   _____

   _____

   _____

2. List three ways in which the LP/VN assists clients in holistic health care.

   (1) _____

   (2) _____

   (3) _____

3. What role does client education play in helping individuals achieve wellness?

   _____

   _____

   _____

4. In what ways does a positive self-concept contribute to an individual's health/wellness?

   _____

   _____

   _____

5. List several healthy behaviors that you practice in your own life.

   (1) _____

   (2) _____

   (3) _____

   (4) _____

   (5) _____

6. How do you deal with anxiety or stress?

   _____

   _____

   _____

7.  What changes would you like to make in your own physical/psychological wellness?

_____

_____

_____

8.  Using the following image, draw a line from the term on the left to the appropriate location on the image.

Love and belonging needs

Physiological needs

Self-actualization needs

Self-esteem needs

Safety and security needs

Courtesy of Delmar Cengage Learning

9.  For each of the preceding levels of need, list two specific ways it would apply to your own life.

**Love and belonging needs**      (1) _____

(2) _____

**Physiological needs**      (1) _____

(2) _____

**Self-actualization needs**      (1) _____

(2) _____

**Self-esteem needs**      (1) _____

(2) _____

**Safety and security needs**      (1) _____

(2) _____

10.  Read the following scenario and answer the questions:

J.W., a 32-year-old paraplegic who runs a small computer consulting business, sought help from a mental health clinic because of recurrent depression. His most recent episode seems to have been precipitated by his girlfriend "dumping" him. Prior to his injury, he was an ambulance driver. His injury occurred 5 years ago in a work-related accident when the ambulance he was driving was hit by a driver who failed to stop at a stop sign. He had been an avid hiker, rock climber, and mountain bike enthusiast prior to his injury. In the past couple of years, he has become involved in a para-basketball league. He was working out at a local gym three times a week until about 6 weeks ago, when the depression worsened.

a.  Using the following blank image, identify the five parts of wellness.

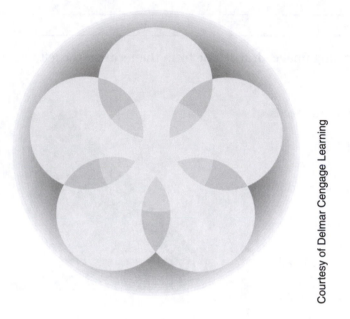

Courtesy of Delmar Cengage Learning

b.  Within each circle, identify the client's issues as they relate to each of the five parts of wellness.

c.  As an LPN/VN, what would your role and responsibilities be regarding the care of this client?

_____

_____

_____

## Self-Assessment Questions

Circle the letter that corresponds to the best answer.

1. Homeostasis can best be described as the
   a. middle range of the health–illness continuum.
   b. integration of holistic modalities into client care.
   c. organism's attempt to balance body, mind, and spirit.
   d. highest level of wellness possible for an individual.

2. The nursing student explains that which is true according to Maslow's Hierarchy of Needs?
   a. Basic physiological needs must be met before higher-level needs.
   b. All physiological and psychosocial needs must be met to maintain life.
   c. An individual moves steadily up the hierarchy toward self-actualization.
   d. Nursing care plans should focus on clients' physiological needs.

3. A client's ability to maintain a positive attitude while being treated for a serious illness is an indication of
   a. self-awareness.
   b. spiritual wellness.
   c. intellectual adaptation.
   d. psychological wellness.

4. The individual whose posture demonstrates good alignment, with shoulders back and head held up, conveys
   a. self-confidence.
   b. aggression.
   c. domination.
   d. curiosity.

5. The most effective way to teach wellness to a client is to
   a. assist the client in developing self-awareness.
   b. be a positive example by practicing good health habits.
   c. explain to the client what can be done to improve health.
   d. explain the concept of wellness in terms the client can understand.

6. An individual's place on the health continuum
   a. does not require constant effort.
   b. can be maintained easily.
   c. demonstrates good physical self-care at a lower level.
   d. can change daily or even hourly.

7. Which of the following needs is not within Maslow's physiological level?
   a. Food
   b. Activity
   c. Shelter
   d. Sex

8. Which of the following best describes self-concept?
   a. It is how others perceive an individual.
   b. It begins forming in infancy.
   c. It is formed solely by negative experiences.
   d. It is not affected during the developing years.

9. One life-cycle consideration for a client's nutritional need is that
   a. proper food choices are more important than quantity of food eaten.
   b. the amount of food eaten increases in the elderly person.
   c. children's appetites do not vary.
   d. healthy eating habits should be established during adulthood.

10. Which of the following best describes spirituality?
    a. It is the concept of religion.
    b. It is not a major healing force.
    c. It involves one's relationship with self, others, the natural order, and a higher power.
    d. It cannot be understood.

# Nursing History, Education, and Organizations

## Key Terms

Match the following terms with their correct definitions.

___ 1. Accreditation

___ 2. Autonomy

___ 3. Clinical

___ 4. Didactic

___ 5. Empowerment

___ 6. Health maintenance organization

___ 7. Morbidity

___ 8. Mortality

___ 9. Nursing

___10. Primary care provider

___11. Primary health care

___12. Staff development

a. Systematic presentation of information.

b. Process by which a voluntary, nongovernmental agency or organization appraises and grants accredited status to institutions and/or programs or services that meet predetermined structure, process, and outcome criteria.

c. Client's point of entry into the health care system; includes assessment, diagnosis, treatment, coordination of care, education, prevention services, and surveillance.

d. Death.

e. Prepaid health plan that provides primary health care services for a preset fee and focuses on cost-effective treatment methods.

f. Delivery of instruction to assist the nurse in achieving the goals of the employer.

g. Illness.

h. Observing and caring for living clients.

i. Health care provider whom a client sees first for health care.

j. An art and a science that assists individuals to learn to care for themselves whenever possible; also involves caring for others when they are unable to meet their own needs.

k. Self-direction.

l. Process of enabling others to do for themselves.

## Abbreviation Review

Write the meaning or definition of the following abbreviations/acronyms.

1. ADN _____

2. *AJN* _____

3. ANA _____

4. APRN _____

5. BSN _____

6. CEPN-LTC _____

7. CEU _____

8. CLTC _____

9. CPNP _____

10. GED _____

11. HMO _____

12. ICN _____

13. JCAHO _____

14. LPN _____

15. LP/VN _____

16. LVN _____

17. NAPNES _____

18. NCLEX _____

19. NCSBN _____

20. NFLPN _____

21. NLN _____

22. NLNAC _____

23. OBRA _____

24. RN _____

25. TEFRA _____

26. USDHHS _____

## Exercises and Activities

1. Describe four nursing leaders who have had a significant impact on nursing and health care.

a. _____

_____

b. _____

_____

c. _____

_____

d. _____

_____

2. Briefly describe how each of these events affected the nursing profession in the United States.

a.  Nightingale's service in Crimea: _____

_____

_____

b.   The founding of the American Red Cross: _____

_____

_____

c.   The founding of the Ballard School: _____

_____

_____

d.   Flexner Report: _____

_____

_____

e.   The establishment of the American Nurses Association: _____

_____

_____

f.   Goldmark Report: _____

_____

_____

g.   The establishment of the National Association for Practical Nurse Education and Service: _

_____

_____

h.   The establishment of insurance plans: _____

_____

_____

i.   Visiting Nurses Associations: _____

_____

_____

j.   Brown Report: _____

_____

_____

k.   The establishment of the National League for Nursing: _____

_____

_____

Insert dates and place each of the preceding events on the following time line:

2003

3. Refer to the Nursing Practice Standards for LPNs (Table 3-2) to decide which of the following topics addresses each activity listed.
   a. Education
   b. Legal/ethical status
   c. Practice
   d. Continuing education
   e. Specialized nursing practice

   _____ Participates in peer review and evaluation processes
   _____ Successfully passes the NCLEX for Practical Nurses
   _____ Does not accept or perform professional activities for which she is not competent
   _____ Applies nursing knowledge and skills to promote health
   _____ Determines new career goals
   _____ Requires completion of at least 1 year's experience in nursing
   _____ Completes an orientation program for employment
   _____ Maintains a current license to practice nursing

## Self-Assessment Questions

Circle the letter that corresponds to the best answer.

1. The process of enabling others to do for themselves is called
   a. competency.
   b. autonomy.
   c. empowerment.
   d. endorsement.

2. Florence Nightingale promoted the use of
   a. public health agencies.
   b. rural nursing services.
   c. nursing organizations.
   d. environmental modifications.

3. The women's rights movement in the 1800s advanced nursing by
   a. supporting university education for women.
   b. effecting federal and state health care legislation.
   c. extending the right to vote to women.
   d. founding professional nursing organizations.

4. Florence Nightingale can be credited with
   a. establishing the Kaiserswerth Institute.
   b. lowering morbidity and mortality rates.
   c. promoting public health nursing.
   d. providing nursing care to indigent people.

5. Which of the following outcomes could be attributed to the Goldmark Report?
   a. Provision of autonomy of practice to home health care nurses
   b. Establishment of nursing research and publications
   c. Identification of inadequacies in nursing education
   d. Enactment of federal funding for nursing education

6. Who organized the Red Cross in the United States?
   a. Dorothea Dix
   b. Clara Barton
   c. Isabel Hampton Robb
   d. Lillian Wald

7. The Mary Mahoney Award is bestowed in recognition of individuals who have made contributions in
   a. nursing leadership.
   b. public health nursing.
   c. nursing education.
   d. improving relationships among cultural groups.

8. Standards for the licensed practical/vocational nurse in legal/ethical status include
   a. knowing the scope of nursing practice.
   b. participating in continuing education activities.
   c. observing, recording, and reporting changes that require intervention.
   d. maintaining the highest possible level of professional competence at all times.

9. Which nursing organization restricts its membership to registered nurses only?
   a. National League for Nursing
   b. National Association for Practical Nurse Education and Service, Inc.
   c. American Nurses Association
   d. National Council of State Boards of Nursing, Inc.

10. Title III of the Health Amendment Act of 1955 resulted in
    a. an alternative to private health insurance.
    b. the establishment of practical nursing.
    c. different levels of nursing.
    d. a deficit in the supply of nurses.

# Legal and Ethical Responsibilities

## Key Terms

Match the following terms with their correct definitions.

_____ 1. Active euthanasia

_____ 2. Administrative law

_____ 3. Advance directive

_____ 4. Assault

_____ 5. Assisted suicide

_____ 6. Autonomy

_____ 7. Battery

_____ 8. Beneficence

_____ 9. Bioethics

_____10. Client advocate

_____11. Civil law

_____12. Confidential

a. Civil wrong committed by a person against another person or property.

b. Wrong that results from a deliberate deception intended to produce unlawful gain.

c. A legal document designating who may make health care decisions for a client when that client is no longer capable of decision making.

d. Law developed by those persons who are appointed to governmental administrative agencies and who are entrusted with enforcing the statutory laws passed by the legislature.

e. Contract that recognizes a relationship between parties for services.

f. Obligation one has incurred or might incur through any act or failure to act.

g. Written instruction for health care that is recognized under state law and is related to the provision of such care when the individual is incapacitated.

h. Situation wherein a person is made to wrongfully believe that he cannot leave a place.

i. Negligent acts on the part of a professional; relates to the conduct of a person who is acting in a professional capacity.

j. Statute that is enacted by the legislature of a state and that outlines the scope of nursing practice in that state.

k. Enforcement of duties and rights among individuals independent of contractual agreements.

l. Laws that provide protection to health care providers by ensuring them immunity from civil liability when care is provided at the scene of an emergency and the caregiver does not intentionally or recklessly cause the client injury.

___13. Constitutional law

___14. Contract law

___15. Criminal law

___16. Defamation

___17. Deontology

___18. Durable power of attorney for health care

___19. Ethical dilemna

___20. Ethical principles

___21. Ethical reasoning

___22. Ethics

___23. Euthanasia

___24. Expressed contract

___25. False imprisonment

___26. Felony

___27. Fidelity

___28. Formal contract

___29. Fraud

___30. Good Samaritan Laws

___31. Impaired nurse

m. Enforcement of agreements among private individuals.

n. Threat to do something that may cause harm or be unpleasant to another person.

o. Written contract that cannot be changed legally by an oral agreement.

p. A competent client's ability to make health care decisions based on full disclosure of the benefits, risks, potential consequences of a recommended treatment plan, and alternate treatments, including no treatment, and the client's agreement to the treatment as indicated by the client's signing a consent form.

q. Risk-management tool used to describe and report any unusual event that occurs to a client, visitor, or staff member.

r. Law that deals with an individual's relationship to the state.

s. Guidelines established to direct nursing care.

t. Unauthorized or unwanted touching of one person by another.

u. Law concerning acts of offense against the welfare or safety of the public.

v. Crime of a serious nature that is usually punishable by imprisonment in a state penitentiary or by death.

w. Conditions and terms of a contract given in writing by the concerned parties.

x. Law that deals with relationships between individuals.

y. Offense that is less serious than a felony and may be punished by a fine or by sentence to a local prison for less than 1 year.

z. Words that are communicated verbally to a third party and that harm or injure the personal or professional reputation of another.

aa. Law enacted by legislative bodies.

bb. Written words that harm or injure the personal or professional reputation of another person.

cc. Private or secret.

dd. Nurse who is habitually intemperate or is addicted to the use of alcohol or habit-forming drugs.

ee. Use of words to harm or injure the personal or professional reputation of another person.

____32. Implied contract

ff. Rehabilitation program that provides an impaired nurse with referrals, professional and peer counseling support groups, and assistance and monitoring to get back into nursing.

____33. Incident report

gg. That which is laid down or fixed.

____34. Informed consent

hh. Law that defines and limits the power of government.

____35. Justice

ii. Any device used to restrict movement.

____36. Law

jj. General term referring to careless acts on the part of an individual who is not exercising reasonable or prudent judgment.

____37. Liability

kk. Legal document that allows a person to state preferences about the use of life-sustaining measures should she be unable to make her wishes known.

____38. Libel

ll. Individual's collection of inner beliefs that guides the way the person acts and helps determine the choices the person makes.

____39. Living will

mm. Application of general ethical principles to health care.

____40. Malpractice

nn. Process of thinking through what one ought to do in an orderly, systematic manner based on principles.

____41. Material principle of justice

oo. Principles that influence the development of beliefs and attitudes.

____42. Misdemeanor

pp. Calling attention to unethical, illegal, or incompetent actions of others.

____43. Negligence

qq. Situation wherein there is a conflict between two or more ethical principles.

____44. Nonmaleficence

rr. Ethical theory that states that the value of a situation is determined by its consequences.

____45. Nursing Practice Act

ss. Process of taking deliberate action that will hasten a client's death.

____46. Passive euthanasia

tt. Branch of philosophy concerned with determining right from wrong on the basis of a body of knowledge.

____47. Peer assistance program

uu. Ethical principle based on the concept of fairness extended to each individual.

____48. Privacy

vv. Person who speaks up for or acts on behalf of the client.

____49. Public law

ww. Situation wherein another person provides a client with the means to end his own life.

____50. Restraint

xx. Ethical principle based on the duty to promote good and prevent harm.

____51. Slander

yy. Process of analyzing one's own values to better understand those things that are truly important.

____52. Standards of practice

zz. Ethical principle that states that an act must result in the greatest degree of good for the greatest number of people involved in a given situation.

___53. Statutory law

   aaa. Ethical principle based on the individual's right to choose and the individual's ability to act on that choice.

___54. Teleology

   bbb. Ethical theory that considers the intrinsic significance of an act as the criterion for determination of good.

___55. Tort

   ccc. Ethical principle based on truthfulness (neither lying to nor deceiving others).

___56. Tort law

   ddd. Widely accepted codes, generally based on the humane aspects of society, that direct or govern actions.

___57. Utility

   eee. Intentional action or lack of action that causes the merciful death of someone suffering from a terminal illness or incurable condition; derived from the Greek word *euthanatos,* which means "good or gentle death."

___58. Value system

   fff. Rationale for determining those times when there can be unequal allocation of scarce resources.

___59. Values

   ggg. Process of cooperating with the client's dying process.

___60. Value clarification

   hhh. Ethical concept based on faithfulness and keeping promises.

___61. Veracity

   iii. Ethical principle based on the obligation to cause no harm to others.

___62. Whistle-blowing

   jjj. The right to be left alone, to choose care based on personal beliefs, to govern body integrity, and to choose how sensitive information is shared.

## Abbreviation Review

Write the meaning or definition of the following abbreviations/acronyms.

1. ADA _____
2. AHA _____
3. AMA _____
4. ANA _____
5. CPR _____
6. DNR _____
7. DPAHC _____
8. ED _____
9. FCA _____
10. HIPAA_____
11. HIPDB _____
12. HIV _____
13. ICN _____
14. IM _____
15. JCAHO _____
16. LP/VN _____

17. NCLEX _____
18. NFLPN _____
19. PHI _____
20. RN _____
21. VA _____

## Exercises and Activities

1. Give examples of how each of the following may directly affect your practice as an LP/VN.

   a. Statutory law: _____
   _____

   b. Administrative law: _____
   _____

   c. Contract law:  _____
   _____

   d. Good Samaritan Acts: _____
   _____

   e. Nursing Practice Act:  _____
   _____

2. Match each situation with the probable type of tort involved.
   a. Assault and battery
   b. False imprisonment
   c. Invasion of privacy
   d. Defamation, libel
   e. Defamation, slander
   f. Negligence
   g. Malpractice

   _____ A student nurse is overheard talking in the cafeteria with fellow students about a client and his recent bout of depression.

   _____ A nurse asks a client why she chose Dr. Smith for her physician, saying, "He treats his patients like they were children and is always so rude to the staff."

   _____ The nurse caring for a client with a new leg cast fails to routinely check the foot for adequate circulation. The client requires additional treatment and loses some function as a result.

   _____ The nurse is preparing to administer an intravenous antibiotic to the client. Because of a failure to check the armband, the wrong client receives the medication.

   _____ The nurse misreads an order for "2u of insulin" as "20 units of insulin," resulting in harm to the client.

   _____ A nurse fails to obtain an order for restraints that were initiated on a client who had become confused.

   _____ A client is told he must pay the remainder of his medical bill before he can leave the facility.

   _____ The names of the clients in a hospital unit are displayed on an assignment board.

   _____ Although the client is showing signs of an adverse reaction to a medication, the physician orders the medication to be continued. The nurse follows the physician's order.

3. Describe correct documentation in terms of timing of the entries, legibility, and thoroughness. In what ways can documentation support a nurse's actions?

   _____

   _____

4. What is the difference between a durable power of attorney for health care and a living will?

   _____

   _____

   _____

   a. Describe in your own words what you might include in your own health care directive or living will. Who would you designate to make health care decisions? What treatments would you want to have withheld?

   _____

   _____

   _____

   b. How is a DNR order different from a living will?

   _____

   _____

   _____

5. P.L. is being treated for a fracture of his right hip. The nurse assigned to care for him is reviewing his chart for information. Because there is no advance directive, the nurse asks P.L. if he would like information or assistance to complete one. P.L. is uncomfortable and tells the nurse to let his wife sign any papers because she is the one who would make the decisions anyway.

   a. How could you explain an advance directive to P.L. and his wife? Can his wife sign the forms for him?

   _____

   _____

   b. P.L. is scheduled for surgery and the nurse is asked to witness the surgical consent form. In what circumstances should the nurse refuse to witness the form?

   _____

   _____

   c. The nurse believes that P.L. does not understand the surgical procedure or the risks involved. What should the nurse do?

   _____

   _____

   d. This nurse was actually assigned to a pediatric unit but was "floated" to P.L.'s unit for the day. The nurse feels unfamiliar with the equipment and medications used with the clients on this unit. What is her responsibility?

   _____

   _____

e. Could the nurse be held liable if P.L. suffers as a result of improper nursing care? How might personal malpractice or liability insurance help the nurse in this situation?

_____

_____

## Exercises and Activities

1. Address the following concerning why ethical dilemmas occur in health care.
   a. Write your values or beliefs about each of the following issues:
   Passive euthanasia: _____

   _____

   Active euthanasia: _____

   _____

   Assisted suicide: _____

   _____

   Refusal of treatment: _____

   _____

   Organ donation and selection of organ recipients: _____

   _____

   b. How is the process of values clarification helpful to you?

   _____

   _____

2. Differentiate each of the following terms:
   a. Ethics vs. values

   _____

   _____

   b. Ethical vs. legal

   _____

   _____

   c. Nonmaleficence vs. negligence

   _____

   _____

   d. Teleology vs. deontology

   _____

   _____

3. Complete each of the following statements:

a. Understanding ethical principles is important for the nurse because _____

_____

b. The nurse bases the care of clients on ethical behavior because _____

_____

c. The Code for Licensed Practical/Vocational Nurses is important because _____

_____

d. If faced with an ethical dilemma, the nurse should _____

_____

4. A.N. gave birth to her fourth child 10 months ago. She received no prenatal care. The baby was diagnosed at birth with a serious genetic disorder that causes severe retardation, facial and skull abnormalities, and heart defects. Survival past a few months of age is rare. A.N. had originally been advised to withhold feedings and allow the infant to die. Instead, she chose to feed and care for her child at home in addition to her other children. Since then, however, A.N. has repeatedly brought the child back to the hospital for medical treatment, at great expense to the hospital. Members of the health care team have asked A.N. to meet with them to discuss her child's medical issues.

a. For this situation, what are the ethical issues involved?

_____

_____

b. In what way are each of the following ethical principles involved?

Autonomy: _____

_____

Nonmaleficence: _____

_____

Justice: _____

_____

Veracity: _____

_____

c. What are the consequences of providing or withholding care?

_____

_____

d. Who should represent the interests of the child in this situation?

_____

e. Should the costs of providing care be a factor in any decisions?

_____

f. What is the nurse's role in this process?

_____

## Self-Assessment Questions

1. An intentional tort differs from an unintentional tort. A nurse fails to verify a questionable order with the physician, resulting in harm to the client. This is an example of
   a. battery.
   b. negligence.
   c. malpractice.
   d. misdemeanor.

2. A client who resides in a facility that receives Medicare funding must
   a. forgo life-prolonging procedures.
   b. complete a living will document.
   c. initiate a durable power of attorney for health care.
   d. have the opportunity to complete an advance directive.

3. An incident or variance report is most useful in any health care institution to help
   a. clarify in the client's chart what happened in an incident.
   b. identify problem areas for possible lawsuits.
   c. prevent a lawsuit from being initiated.
   d. document poor professional activities.

4. A nurse is asked by a neighbor to look at her child who is ill. In this situation, the nurse would be
   a. liable for any harm caused by misdiagnosis or treatment.
   b. protected by his employer's liability policy.
   c. protected by the Good Samaritan Act.
   d. violating the Nursing Practice Act.

5. The first priority for the nurse who suspects a colleague is using habit-forming drugs is to
   a. determine what laws may have been broken.
   b. document any incidences and report to a supervisor.
   c. report the colleague to the State Board of Nursing.
   d. confront the colleague with any suspicions.

6. The ethical foundation of the nurse–client relationship is the
   a. duty to promote good and prevent harm.
   b. principle of nonmaleficence.
   c. Patient's Bill of Rights.
   d. concept of fidelity.

7. The principle that an act must result in the greatest degree of good for the greatest number of people involved in a given situation is called
   a. utility.
   b. beneficence.
   c. client advocacy.
   d. situational theory.

8. The Patient's Bill of Rights is most useful
   a. to guide health care workers in treatment decisions.
   b. to outline clients' responsibilities and ways they will be treated in the hospital.
   c. as a legally binding contract between health care workers and clients.
   d. to provide a framework for ethical dilemmas.

9. If you are caring for a client whose value system conflicts with your own, you should first attempt to
   a. be aware of your own values.
   b. ask the client to clarify her values.
   c. engage in a meaningful dialogue with the client.
   d. determine which nursing actions you are willing to do.

10. The first step in ethical decision making is to
    a. examine the values involved.
    b. recognize the ethical dimension of the issue.
    c. discuss the issue with relevant others.
    d. check the legal and organizational policies.

# The Health Care Delivery System

## Key Terms

Match the following terms with their correct definitions.

___ 1. Capitated rate

___ 2. Comorbidity

___ 3. Exclusive provider organization

___ 4. Fee-for-Service

___ 5. Health care delivery system

___ 6. Health maintenance organization

___ 7. Managed care

___ 8. Medicaid

___ 9. Medical model

___10. Medicare

___11. Medigap insurance

___12. Preferred provider organization

a. Simultaneous existence of more than one disease process within an individual.

b. System of providing and monitoring care wherein access, cost, and quality are controlled before or during delivery of services.

c. Care focused on promoting wellness and preventing illness.

d. Preset fee based on membership rather than services provided; payment system used in managed care.

e. Organization wherein care must be delivered by the plan in order for clients to receive reimbursement for health care services.

f. Health care provider whom a client sees first for health care, typically a family practitioner (physician/nurse), internist, or pediatrician.

g. Predetermined rate paid for each episode of hospitalization based on the client's age and principal diagnosis and the presence or absence of surgery or comorbidity.

h. Health care delivery model wherein the government is the only entity to reimburse.

i. Prepaid health plan that provides primary health car services for a preset fee and focuses on cost-effective treatment methods.

j. System in which the health care recipient directly pays the provider for services as they are provided.

k. Traditional approach to health care wherein the focus is on treatment and cure of disease.

l. Legal recognition of the ability to prescribe medications.

____13. Prescriptive authority

____14. Primary care

____15. Primary care provider

____16. Primary health care

____17. Prospective payment

____18. Secondary care

____19. Single-payer system

____20. Single point of entry

____21. Tertiary care

m. Care focused on diagnosis and treatment after the client exhibits symptoms of illness.

n. Plan that covers inpatient hospital care, home health care, and hospice care for individuals over the age of 65, as well as those who are permanently disabled and those with end-stage renal disease.

o. Client's point of entry into the health care system; includes assessment, diagnosis, treatment, coordination of care, education, preventive services, and surveillance.

p. Mechanism for providing services that meet the health-related needs of individuals.

q. Type of managed care model wherein member choice is limited to providers within the system.

r. A common feature of health maintenance organizations wherein the client is required to enter the health care system through a point designated by the plan.

s. Care focused on restoring the client to the state of health that existed before the development of an illness; if unattainable, then care directed to attaining the optimal level of health possible.

t. Pays for health services for low-income families with dependent children, the aged poor, and the disabled.

u. Policies purchased from private insurance companies to pay for costs not covered by Medicare.

## Abbreviation Review

Write the meaning or definition of the following abbreviations/acronyms.

1. ADAMHA _____
2. AHCPR _____
3. AHRQ _____
4. AIDS _____
5. AMA _____
6. ANA _____
7. APRN _____
8. ATSDR _____
9. CDC _____
10. CHIP _____
11. CNM _____
12. CNO _____
13. CNS _____

14. DDS _____

15. DMD _____

16. DRG _____

17. EPO _____

18. FDA _____

19. HCFA _____

20. HMO _____

21. HRSA _____

22. IHS _____

23. LP/VN _____

24. MD _____

25. NFLPN _____

26. NIH _____

27. NLN _____

28. NP _____

29. OT _____

30. PA _____

31. PCP _____

32. PPO _____

33. PT _____

34. RD _____

35. RN _____

36. RPh _____

37. RT _____

38. SW _____

39. USDHHS _____

40. USPHS _____

41. VA _____

## Exercises and Activities

1. What factors have contributed to the increased number of clients now receiving care in outpatient clinics and in-home settings?

   _____

   _____

   _____

2. Explain the nursing roles of:

   a. Caregiver: _____

   _____

b. Teacher: _____

_____

c. Advocate: _____

_____

d. Team member: _____

_____

3. L.C. is a 73-year-old client in your long-term care facility. She was admitted 2 weeks ago to continue her recovery from a hip fracture. Prior to her injury, she had been living alone in a small
apartment in a retirement community not far from her married daughter. She rejects her daughter's offer to move into their home but is now willing to accept some help with cleaning and cooking if it allows her to remain independent.

List activities or referrals for L.C. that would be examples of each level of care.

Primary care: _____

_____

Secondary care: _____

_____

Tertiary care: _____

_____

## Self-Assessment Questions

Circle the letter that corresponds to the best answer.

1. While participating in an immunization clinic for influenza, the nurse is providing
   a. primary care.
   b. secondary care.
   c. tertiary care.
   d. early intervention.

2. The system for financing health care services in the United States is based on
   a. a single-payer system.
   b. a managed care model.
   c. an exclusive provider model.
   d. a private insurance model.

3. The primary goal of managed care is to
   a. provide preventive services by a primary care provider.
   b. provide health education and disease prevention services to clients.
   c. deliver service in the most cost-efficient manner possible.
   d. set fees and determine reasonable reimbursement for medical and surgical treatment.

4. Conducting research and education related to specific diseases is a function of the
   a. Agency for Health Care Policy and Research.
   b. Centers for Disease Control and Prevention.
   c. National Institutes of Health.
   d. Health Resources and Services Administration.

5. The nurse providing care in the hospital setting knows that as a result of the Prospective Payment System and diagnosis-related groups
   a. clients may be discharged sooner.
   b. clients' response to treatment is less important.
   c. clients are less likely to be critically ill.
   d. clients are receiving higher-quality care.

6. A major challenge facing the U.S. health care system is the
   a. lack of prescriptive authority for advanced-practice nurses.
   b. decreased use of hospitals and its impact on quality of care.
   c. greater availability of outpatient facilities and services.
   d. cultural beliefs of a diverse population and their effect on health care.

7. Which health care team member works with clients who have functional impairments and teaches skills for activities of daily living?
   a. Physician's assistant
   b. Social worker
   c. Physical therapist
   d. Occupational therapist

8. Which role is *not* a nursing role?
   a. Caregiver
   b. Therapist
   c. Teacher
   d. Manager

9. A cultural belief or value that may prevent an individual from seeking health care is
   a. refusal of care on holy days.
   b. that illness is a result of sins committed in a previous life.
   c. that one should trust in divine healing.
   d. any of the above.

10. A trend affecting delivery of health care service is
    a. an aging U.S. population.
    b. a decreasing number of single-parent families.
    c. fewer states using managed care to provide services.
    d. a diminished interest in quality improvement.

# Arenas of Care

## Key Terms

Match the following terms with their correct definitions.

___ 1. Accreditation

___ 2. Adult day care

___ 3. Assisted living

___ 4. Certification

___ 5. Hospice

___ 6. Licensure

___ 7. Long-term care facility

___ 8. Rehabilitation

___ 9. Respite care

___10. Subacute care

a. Voluntary process that establishes and evaluates standards of care; mandatory for any health care service receiving federal funds.

b. Process by which a voluntary, nongovernmental agency or organization appraises and grants accredited status to institutions and/or programs or services that meet predetermined structure, process, and outcome criteria.

c. Mandatory system of granting licenses according to specified standards.

d. Process designed to assist individuals to reach their optimal level of physical, mental, and psychosocial functioning.

e. Care and service that provides time off to caregivers and is utilized for a few hours a week, an occasional weekend, or longer periods of time.

f. Humane, compassionate care provided to clients who can no longer benefit from curative treatment and have 6 months or less to live.

g. Combination of housing and services for people who require assistance with activities of daily living.

h. Health care facility that provides services to individuals who are not acutely ill, have continuing health care needs, and cannot function independently at home.

i. Provision of a variety of services in a protective setting for adults who are unable to stay alone but who do not need 24-hour care.

j. Health care designed to provide services for clients who are out of the acute stage of illness but still require skilled nursing, monitoring, and ongoing treatments.

## Abbreviation Review

Write the meaning or definition of the following abbreviations/acronyms.

1. ADL _____
2. AHCA _____
3. AIDS _____
4. ALFA _____
5. APRN _____
6. CARF _____
7. CCRC _____
8. CCU _____
9. CEPN-LTC™ _____
10. CHAP _____
11. CLTC _____
12. CT _____
13. ECF _____
14. ECG _____
15. ED _____
16. EEG _____
17. EMG _____
18. HCFA _____
19. HMO _____
20. IADL _____
21. ICF _____
22. ICU _____
23. IHCT _____
24. JCAHO _____
25. MRI _____
26. OBRA _____
27. OR _____
28. RPCH _____
29. RR _____
30. SBC _____
31. SNF _____

## Exercises and Activities

1. List and explain three nonacute health care services.

_____

_____

_____

2. List several "rights" provided by the resident's rights document that directly affect your nursing care of clients in long-term care facilities.

    (1) _____

    (2) _____

    (3) _____

    (4) _____

    (5) _____

    (6) _____

3. How would you compare Medicare and Medicaid for the type of assistance they provide?

_____

_____

_____

4. Describe the goal of rehabilitation for the client. When does rehabilitation begin?

_____

_____

_____

5. What skills are important for the nurse working in the field of rehabilitation?

_____

_____

_____

6. Identify services that might be used in home health care for the client or family.

_____

_____

_____

7. What are the nurse's responsibilities in the home health care setting?

_____

_____

_____

8. Compare each of the following types of assistance for clients.

    Extended-care facility: _____

    _____

    Subacute care:_____

    _____

    Assisted living:_____

    _____

    Respite care: _____

    _____

Adult day care: _____

_____

Hospice: _____

_____

10. T.P. is a 38-year-old insurance agent who enjoys writing short stories as a hobby. Last week during a storm, a car coming toward him crossed into his lane, hitting him head-on. T. P. was tossed around in the car and thrown out through the windshield. Rescue workers arrived and transported him to the trauma center. After stabilization of the injury and further assessment, it was determined that T. P. had sustained a T8 injury and is paraplegic. Next week he will be transferred to a rehabilitation facility with a spinal cord injury program. An IHCT will focus on assisting T.P. to regain as much independence as possible.

a. Describe the importance of the IHCT for this client in rehabilitation.

_____

_____

_____

b. How would the nurse function as a member of this team?

_____

_____

_____

_____

c. Why is the early assessment and intervention of psychological well-being essential in the rehabilitation process?

_____

_____

_____

_____

d. How can the nurse and the IHCT support T. P.'s efforts toward independence?

_____

_____

_____

_____

e. One month after his transfer to rehabilitation, T. P. appears to be doing well. He has some function of his upper body, including his hands. His immediate learning needs are a.m. care, feeding and grooming, intermittent self-catheterization, and bowel training. List several long-term goals for this client.

(1) _____

(2) _____

(3) _____

(4) _____

(5) _____

f. Why will good nutrition and skin care be lifelong issues for this client?

_____

_____

_____

_____

g. T. P. has limited insurance coverage for the rehabilitation facility. He is now being discharged home and will be seen as an outpatient for 3 hours a day. He is divorced, and he will be moving into his parents' home at least until he has completed his rehabilitation program. How can home health care support his transition to independence?

_____

_____

_____

_____

_____

_____

## Self-Assessment Questions

Circle the letter that corresponds to the best answer.

1. In what setting is hospice care not provided?
   a. Rehabilitation
   b. Acute care
   c. Home care
   d. Outpatient care

2. A home health care nurse has been assigned to care for a client with a chronic illness following discharge from the hospital. A major priority for this nurse will be to
   a. educate the client and family.
   b. maintain accurate documentation.
   c. obtain Medicare/Medicaid funding.
   d. determine the most appropriate placement for long-term care.

3. A primary effect of the Omnibus Budget Reconciliation Act of 1987 on long-term care was to
   a. determine funding for long-term care facilities.
   b. regulate the reporting of client abuse.
   c. provide accreditation for long-term care facilities.
   d. develop the resident's rights document.

4. The increase in nonacute health care services over the past 10 years is related to all but which of the following factors?
    a. Change in costs of health care
    b. Decline in hospital-bed availability
    c. Longer life span of clients with health problems
    d. Early discharge of clients from acute care settings

5. A 68-year-old widowed client, who has just had abdominal surgery for cancer, is expected to do well. There are no family members able to care for the client following early discharge. The most appropriate short-term placement for this client is
    a. hospice.
    b. respite care.
    c. subacute care.
    d. assisted living.

6. All are examples of resident's rights except
    a. right to vote.
    b. right to choose an attending physician.
    c. right to limited access to family of relatives.
    d. right to remain in the facility except in certain circumstances.

7. A voluntary process that indicates that the delivery of care and services is above minimum standards is called
    a. accreditation.
    b. certification.
    c. licensure.
    d. compliance.

8. Health care facilities must be _____ to be reimbursed by government funds, Medicare, and Medicaid.
    a. accredited
    b. certified
    c. licensed
    d. compliant

9. A facility designed to provide services for clients who are out of the acute stage of their illness but still require ongoing treatments, skilled nursing, and monitoring is called
    a. a nursing home.
    b. an adult day care center.
    c. a rest home.
    d. a subacute care facility.

10. Higher-level tasks such as household and money management are part of
    a. ADLs.
    b. PROM.
    c. IADLs.
    d. respite care.

# Communication

## Chapter 7

## Key Terms

Match the following terms with their correct definitions.

_____ 1. Active listening

_____ 2. Aphasia

_____ 3. Communication

_____ 4. Congruent

_____ 5. Dysarthria

_____ 6. Dysphasia

_____ 7. Empathy

_____ 8. Feedback

_____ 9. Hearing

_____10. Interpersonal communication

_____11. Intrapersonal communication

_____12. Listening

_____13. Nonverbal communication

_____14. Professional boundaries

_____15. Proxemics

_____16. Rapport

_____17. Shift report

a. The limits of the professional relationship that allow for a safe, therapeutic connection between the professional and the client.

b. Permits physicians to provide care through a telecommunication system.

c. Communication that is purposeful and goal directed, creating a beneficial outcome for the client.

d. Sending a message without words; sometimes called body language.

e. Difficult and defective speech due to a dysfunction of the muscles used for speech.

f. Response from the receiver of a message so that the sender can verify the message.

g. Process of hearing spoken words and noting nonverbal behaviors.

h. Use of communications technology to transmit health information from one location to another.

i. Using words, either spoken or written, to send a message.

j. Interpreting the sounds heard and attaching meaning to them.

k. Relationship of mutual trust and understanding.

l. Impairment of speech resulting from damage to the speech center in the brain.

m. The sending and receiving of a message.

n. Study of the space between people and its effect on interpersonal behavior.

o. Act or power of receiving sounds.

p. Inability to communicate, as a result of a brain lesion.

q. Agreement between two things.

____18. Telehealth

____19. Telemedicine

____20. Telenursing

____21. Therapeutic communication

____22. Verbal communication

r. Capacity to understand another person's feelings or perception of a situation.

s. Report about each client between shifts.

t. Permits nurses to provide care through a telecommunication system.

u. Self-talk of internal thoughts and discussions with oneself.

v. Basic level of communicating between nurse and client.

## Abbreviation Review

Write the meaning or definition of the following abbreviations.

1. ANA_____.
2. CPR _____
3. HIV _____
4. IOM _____
5. WPM _____

## Exercises and Activities

1. Look at each of these photographs and describe what types of nonverbal communication are present.
   a. Are they positive or negative?

   _____
   _____
   _____
   _____
   _____
   _____
   _____
   _____
   _____

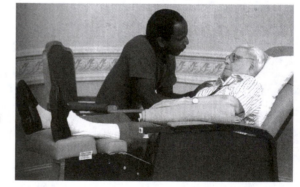

Courtesy of Delmar Cengage Learning

b. What nonverbal communication does the nurse convey?

_____

_____

_____

_____

_____

_____

_____

_____

_____

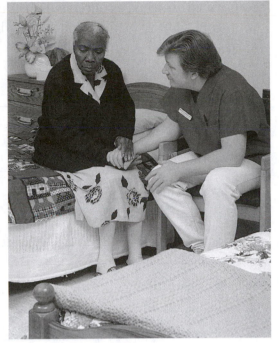

Courtesy of Delmar Cengage Learning

c. What nonverbal communication do you observe in this client?

_____

_____

_____

_____

_____

_____

_____

_____

_____

_____

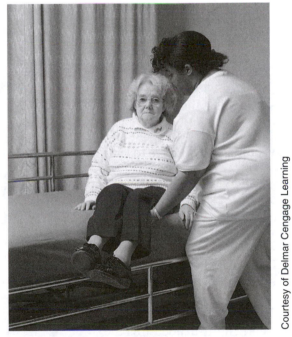

Courtesy of Delmar Cengage Learning

2.  If you were having a conversation with a client right now, how might each of the following factors influence your communication style?

   a.  Your age: _____

   _____

   b.  Your education: _____

   _____

   c.  Your emotions: _____

   _____

   d.  Your culture: _____

   _____

   e.  Your language: _____

   _____

   f.  Your attention: _____

   _____

   g.  Your surroundings: _____

   _____

3.  For each of the following statements, give the communication technique being demonstrated. Does it have a positive or a negative effect? If it is negative, rewrite it in a way that might be therapeutic.

| *Nurse's Statement* | *Technique or Barrier Demonstrated* | *Rewrite If Necessary* |
| --- | --- | --- |
| a. "Tell me about your surgery last month." | | |
| b. "You know the rules about visitors. They'll have to leave." | | |
| c. "Well, I don't believe you should be doing that in your condition." | | |
| d. "You look uncomfortable. Do you need more pain medication?" | | |
| e. "Earlier you talked about feeling light-headed. Tell me more about that." | | |
| f. "Every cloud has a silver lining." | | |
| g. "Under the circumstances, it was the only thing you could do." | | |
| h. "What did you learn in the class this morning?" | | |

4. V.S. is a 42-year-old client recently diagnosed with lung cancer. He is facing surgery tomorrow and appears very worried. At home, his wife is caring for their two children, ages 11 and 14. When you enter his room at the start of your shift, he is sitting quietly in bed and doesn't seem to hear you.

   a. What behaviors or attitudes might help you to communicate with V.S. in a caring manner?

   _____

   _____

   b. How could you begin a conversation with him using one or more of the therapeutic communication techniques?

   _____

   _____

   c. How could you use silence in this situation?

   _____

   _____

## Self-Assessment Questions

Circle the letter that corresponds to the best answer.

1. The nurse caring for a client states, "A minute ago, you said you were sleeping poorly at night. Could you tell me more about that?" This is an example of
   a. reflecting.
   b. restating.
   c. focusing.
   d. paraphrasing.

2. The nurse practicing therapeutic communication will avoid
   a. giving advice.
   b. procedural touch.
   c. using gestures.
   d. silence.

3. The goals of therapeutic communication include
   a. self-disclosure, validation, and empathy.
   b. obtaining information, developing trust, and showing caring.
   c. offering assistance, showing acceptance, and reducing communication blocks.
   d. active listening, data gathering, and developing a communication style.

4. Imposing a personal set of values while caring for a client is a barrier to communication that is called
   a. value sharing.
   b. validating.
   c. giving advice.
   d. judgmental response.

5. To communicate with a client with dysphasia, the nurse will remember to
   a. speak normally.
   b. use slightly exaggerated word formation.
   c. ask a family member to assist.
   d. touch the client's arm before speaking.

6. During a conversation, a client reveals to you that she may be in an abusive relationship. As the nurse, you realize that
   a. you can demonstrate caring by encouraging the client to share her fears.
   b. nurse–client communication is privileged and should be kept confidential.
   c. a client care conference will help determine what steps the client should take.
   d. you have a responsibility to share the information with health care team members.

7. All are forms of verbal communication except
   a. speaking.
   b. listening.
   c. writing.
   d. tone of voice.

8. The statement "Don't worry, I'm sure everything will be fine" is an example of
   a. a cliché.
   b. false reassurance.
   c. belittling.
   d. defending.

9. The statement "Yes, everyone feels like that" is an example of
   a. a cliché.
   b. false reassurance.
   c. belittling.
   d. defending.

10. A person whose style of communication puts his own feelings, needs, and rights first is using a style best described as
    a. aggressive.
    b. assertive.
    c. passive.
    d. judgmental.

# Client Teaching

## Key Terms

Match the following terms with their correct definitions.

___ 1. Affective domain

___ 2. Auditory learner

___ 3. Cognitive domain

___ 4. Formal teaching

___ 5. Informal teaching

___ 6. Kinesthetic learner

___ 7. Learning

___ 8. Learning plateau

___ 9. Learning style

___10. Motivation

___11. Psychomotor domain

___12. Readiness for learning

___13. Self-efficacy

___14. Teaching

___15. Teaching-learning process

a. Planned interaction that promotes a behavioral change that is not a result of maturation or coincidence.

b. Technique to promote learning.

c. Teaching that takes place any time, any place, and whenever a learning need is identified.

d. Area of learning that involves performance of motor skills.

e. Person who learns by processing information through seeing.

f. Belief in one's ability to succeed in attempts to change behavior.

g. Area of learning that involves attitudes, beliefs, and emotions.

h. Teaching that takes place at a specific time, in a specific place, and on a specific topic.

i. Peak in the effectiveness of teaching and depth of learning.

j. Active process wherein one individual shares information with another as a means to facilitate learning and thereby promote behavioral changes.

k. Person who learns by processing information through hearing.

l. Person who learns by processing information through touching, feeling, and doing.

m. Area of learning that involves intellectual understanding.

n. Process of assimilating information, resulting in behavioral change.

o. Evidence of willingness to learn.

___16. Teaching strategy

p. Manner whereby an individual incorporates new information.

___17. Visual learner

q. Forces acting on or within organisms that initiate, direct, or maintain behavior.

## Abbreviation Review

Write the meaning or definition of the following abbreviations.

1. AEB _____
2. JCAHO _____
3. NPO _____
4. R/T _____

## Exercises and Activities

1. Describe the role that client teaching plays to help you provide nursing care.

   _____

   _____

   _____

   How are formal and informal teaching different? Give an example of each.

   _____

   _____

   _____

2. Give examples from your own nursing education program for each of the three learning domains.

   a. Cognitive: _____

   _____

   b. Affective: _____

   _____

   c. Psychomotor: _____

   _____

3. You have been assigned to care for G.R., a 68-year-old woman who was diagnosed with breast cancer. She is now in the hospital recovering from surgery to remove her right breast tissue and lymph nodes. She will need to perform exercises at home to promote healing and maintain circulation and function in her right arm. As you are caring for her, you note that she has a hearing loss and understands some English, but is not fluent. G.R. shares a semiprivate room with another client, and you note that they both have a lot of visitors. One of the visitors is G.R.'s sister, who will be helping her at home during her recovery.

   a. In what ways will your teaching be important to G.R.?

   _____

   _____

b.  How would you determine her readiness to learn?

_____

_____

c.  Write in the following diagram what learning barriers might be present for G.R. Give two interventions that might help overcome each type of learning barrier.

| Type of Barrier | Findings | Interventions |
| --- | --- | --- |
| **External Barriers** | | |
| Environmental | | |
| Sociocultural | | |
| **Internal Barriers** | | |
| Psychological | | |
| Physiological | | |

4.  You have decided that G.R. will need to know how to perform the exercises at home after she is discharged.

a.  What are her specific learning needs?

_____

_____

b.  What types of teaching methods could you use?

_____

_____

c.  List two ways you can evaluate whether G.R. has learned this skill.

(1) _____

(2) _____

d.  Unfortunately, G.R. is having difficulty remembering how you demonstrated the exercises. She appears frustrated and tired. List three ideas that you could use to help with her learning.

(1) _____

(2) _____

(3) _____

e.  Why would it be helpful to discuss community resources with G.R.?

_____

_____

# Self-Assessment Questions

Circle the letter that corresponds to the best answer.

1. In today's health care setting, a major goal of client teaching is to
   a. facilitate and enhance the nurse–client relationship.
   b. assess for psychological and physiological barriers to learning.
   c. determine which clients will benefit most from teaching.
   d. promote wellness and prevent illness.

2. The nurse is teaching a new mother breastfeeding techniques. Which of the following teaching strategies will promote learning in the affective domain?
   a. The nurse determines how much the client already knows about breastfeeding.
   b. The nurse has the client demonstrate how to hold her newborn for feeding.
   c. The nurse encourages the client to discuss her family's attitude toward breastfeeding.
   d. The client explains why breast milk is the most beneficial for her newborn.

3. When teaching a client who is hearing impaired, an effective approach would include
   a. using repetition of the materials.
   b. providing large-print education materials.
   c. using short sentences and words that are easily understood.
   d. determining the client's self-care abilities.

4. Client teaching is mandated by JCAHO and the Patient's Bill of Rights because
   a. informed consent is essential to health care.
   b. more patients are being discharged sooner from hospitals.
   c. an educated client is able to achieve higher levels of wellness.
   d. the client develops positive feelings toward health care providers.

5. Which of the following teaching methods would promote learning in the cognitive domain?
   a. Demonstration and supervised practice
   b. Games and computer activities
   c. Discussion and role play
   d. Visual stimuli and return demonstration

6. Formal teaching includes
   a. instruction on a specific topic, at a specific time.
   b. unscripted answers to a question.
   c. explaining the care being given to a client at the time of care.
   d. instruction at any time or place.

7. That clients must believe that they need to learn the information before learning can occur is an example of which learning principle?
   a. Maturation
   b. Readiness
   c. Motivation
   d. Relevance

8. That clients should be able and willing to learn is an example of which learning principle?
   a. Maturation
   b. Readiness
   c. Motivation
   d. Relevance

9. Retention of material is reinforced by
   a. checking literacy.
   b. maturation.
   c. organization.
   d. repetition.

10. The visual learner would prefer information in the form of
    a. question-and-answer sessions.
    b. handouts.
    c. lectures.
    d. discussion sessions.

# Nursing Process/ Documentation/Informatics

## Key Terms

Match the following terms with their correct definitions.

_o_ 1. Actual nursing diagnosis

____ 2. Analysis

____ 3. Assessment

____ 4. Assessment model

_a_ 5. Charting by exception

____ 6. Comprehensive assessment

____ 7. Critical pathway

____ 8. Data clustering

____ 9. Defining characteristics

____10. Dependent nursing intervention

____11. Discharge planning

____12. Documentation

_d_ 13. Etiology

a. Continuous updating of the client's plan of care.

b. Review of the client's functional health patterns prior to the current contact with the health care agency.

c. Process of putting data together in order to identify areas of the client's problems and strengths.

d. Cause of or contributor to a problem.

e. Written guide that organizes data about a client's care into a formal statement of the strategies that will be implemented to help the client achieve optimal health.

f. Order written in a client's medical record or nursing care plan by a physician or nurse especially for that individual client; not used for any other client.

g. Putting data together in a new way.

h. Clinical judgment by the physician that identifies or determines a specific disease, condition, or pathological state.

i. Fifth step in the nursing process; involves determining whether client goals have been met, partially met, or not met.

j. Second step in the nursing process; a clinical judgment about individual, family, or community (aggregate) responses to actual or potential health problems/life processes.

k. Nursing diagnosis that indicates the client's expression of a desire to obtain a higher level of wellness in some area of function; composed of the diagnostic label preceded by the phrase "potential for enhanced."

l. Data source other than the client; can include family members, other health care providers, or medical records.

m. Fourth step in the nursing process; involves the execu-

___14. Evaluation

___15. Expected outcome

___16. Focus charting

___17. Focused assessment

___18. Goal

___19. Health history

___20. Implementation

___21. Incident report

___22. Independent nursing intervention

___23. Initial planning

___24. Interdependent nursing intervention

___25. Kardex

___26. Long-term goal

___27. Medical diagnosis

___28. Narrative charting

___29. Nursing care plan

tion of the nursing plan of care formulated during the planning phase.

n. Framework that provides a systematic method for organizing data.

o. Nursing diagnosis that indicates that a problem exists; composed of the diagnostic label, related factors, and signs and symptoms.

p. Planning that involves critical anticipation and planning for the client's needs after discharge.

q. Nursing action that is implemented in a collaborative manner with other health care professionals.

r. Observable and measurable data that are obtained through standard assessment techniques performed during the physical examination and through laboratory and diagnostic tests.

s. Type of assessment that is limited in scope in order to focus on a particular need or health care problem or on potential health care risks.

t. Third step of the nursing process; includes both the formulation of guidelines that establish the proposed course of nursing action in the resolution of nursing diagnoses and the development of the client's plan of care.

u. First step in the nursing process; includes systematic collection, verification, organization, interpretation, and documentation of data.

v. Type of assessment that includes systematic monitoring and observation related to specific problems.

w. Comprehensive, standard plan of care for specific case situations.

x. Nursing action that requires an order from a physician or other health care professional.

y. Major provider of information about a client.

z. Objective that outlines the desired resolution of the nursing diagnosis over a short period of time, usually a few hours or days (less than a week).

aa. Elements that should be in clinical records and abstracted for studies on the effectiveness and costs of nursing care.

bb. Collected data; also known as signs and symptoms, subjective and objective data, or clinical manifestations.

cc. Action performed by a nurse that helps the client achieve the results specified by the goals and expected outcomes.

___30. Nursing diagnosis

dd. Standardized intervention written, approved, and signed by a physician that is kept on file within health care agencies to be used in predictable situations or in circumstances requiring immediate attention.

___31. Nursing intervention

ee. Development of a preliminary plan of care by the nurse who performs the admission assessment and gathers the comprehensive admission assessment data.

___32. Nursing Intervention Classification (NIC)

ff. Type of assessment that provides baseline client data, including a complete health history and current needs assessment.

___33. Nursing Minimum Data Set (NMDS)

gg. Detailed, specific statement that describes the methods through which a goal will be achieved and that includes aspects such as direct nursing care, client teaching, and continuity of care.

___34. Nursing Outcomes Classification (NOC)

hh. Objective that outlines the desired resolution of the nursing diagnosis over a longer period of time, usually weeks or months.

___35. Nursing process

ii. Nursing diagnosis indicating that a problem does not yet exist but that specific risk factors are present; composed of the diagnostic label followed by the phrase "Risk for" and a list of the specific risk factors.

___36. Objective data

jj. Statement written in objective format and demonstrating an expectation to be achieved in resolution of the nursing diagnosis over a long period of time, usually weeks or months.

___37. Ongoing assessment

kk. Data from the client's point of view, including feelings, perceptions, and concerns.

___38. Ongoing planning

ll. Systematic method of providing care to clients, consisting of five steps: assessment, diagnosis, outcome identification and planning, implementation, and evaluation.

___39. PIE charting

mm. Breaking down the whole into parts that can be examined.

___40. Planning

nn. Nursing action initiated by the nurse that does not require direction or an order from another health care professional.

___41. Point-of-care charting

oo. Written evidence of the interactions between and among health care professionals, clients and their families, and health care organizations; the administration of tests, procedures, treatments, and client education; and the result of or client's response to diagnostic tests and interventions.

___42. Primary source

pp. Standardized language for nursing outcomes.

_55_ 43. Problem-oriented medical record

qq. Documentation of an unusual occurrence or an accident in delivery of client care.

___44. Risk nursing diagnosis

rr. Documentation method that requires the nurse to document only deviations from preestablished norms.

_1_45. Secondary source

ss. Documentation method focusing on the client's problem and using a structured, logical format to narrative charting, categorized by subjective data, objective data, assessment, and plan.

___46. Short-term goal

tt. Reporting method used when members of the care team walk to each client's room and discuss care with each other and with the client.

___47. SOAP charting

uu. Goals not met or interventions not performed according to the time frame; also called variances.

_ZZ_48. Source-oriented charting

vv. Documentation system that allows health care providers to gain immediate access to client information at the bedside.

___49. Specific order

ww. Standardized language for nursing interventions.

___50. Standing order

xx. Documentation method using a column format to chart data, actions, and responses.

___51. Subjective data

yy. Documentation method using the problem, intervention, evaluation format.

___52. Synthesis

zz. Narrative recording by each member (source) of the health care team on a separate record.

___53. Variance

aaa. Documentation method using subjective data, objective data, assessment, and plan.

___54. Walking rounds

bbb. Summary worksheet reference of basic client care information.

___55. Wellness nursing diagnosis

ccc. Story format of documentation that describes the client's status, the interventions and treatments, and the client's response to treatments.

# Abbreviation Review

Write the meaning or definition of the following abbreviations, acronyms, and symbols.

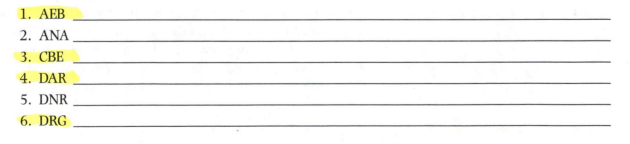

1. AEB _____

2. ANA _____

3. CBE _____

4. DAR _____

5. DNR _____

6. DRG _____

   7. HIS _____

   8. JCAHO _____

   9. L _____

10. MAR _____

11. NANDA _____

12. NIC _____

13. NIS _____

14. NMDS _____

15. NOC _____

16. PIE _____

17. POMR _____

18. PPS _____

19. PRO _____

20. RN _____

21. ROM _____

22. R/T _____

23. SOAP _____

24. SOAPIE _____

25. SOAPIER _____

26. t.o. _____

27. UMLS _____

## Exercises and Activities

1. Write a short definition for each phase of the nursing process: Assessment, Planning, Intervention, and Evaluation.

   _____

   _____

   _____

   _____

2. Differentiate the three types of nursing diagnoses: actual, risk (potential problem), and wellness.

   _____

   _____

   _____

   _____

   a.  How does a three-part statement of a diagnosis differ from a two-part statement?

   _____

   _____

b.  Give one example of a two-part statement for each type of nursing diagnosis.

Actual: _____

Risk (potential problem): _____

Wellness: _____

3.  In what ways does a nursing diagnosis differ from a medical diagnosis?

_____

_____

a.  For each of the following medical diagnoses, write two nursing diagnoses that might apply to a client.

| Medical Diagnosis | Nursing Diagnosis |
|---|---|
| Myocardial infarction | (1) _____ |
| | (2) _____ |
| Anorexia | (1) _____ |
| | (2) _____ |
| Fracture of the pelvis | (1) _____ |
| | (2) _____ |

b.  Choose one of your nursing diagnoses from the preceding table and write it as a three-part statement.

_____

_____

4.  Where do you find each of these items in a nursing care plan?
   a.  Assessment
   b.  Diagnoses
   c.  Planning and outcome identification
   d.  Implementation
   e.  Evaluation

_____  "Take blood pressure every 3 hours."

_____  "Instruct client to self-administer medication."

_____  "Exercises three times a week to relieve stress."

_____  "I have been having headaches for the past week."

_____  "Client will eat 75% of meal with assistance."

_____  "Vitals signs will remain stable."

_____  "Anxiety related to hospitalization."

_____  "Sleep pattern disturbance."

_____  "Assess and document patient's sleeping pattern."

_____  "Goal met: client able to select appropriate foods for low-sodium diet."

_____  "Client was able to state signs and symptoms of infection."

5. Review the following client health history. O.N. was diagnosed 2 years ago with type II diabetes and takes metformin (Glucophage) 500 mg b.i.d. (twice a day) with meals. She is being seen in the clinic for her 6-month visit. She says, "I hardly have the energy to get up and dress in the morning. I am thirsty all day and awaken several times during the night, having to go to the bathroom." She does not work outside the home and has not been involved in community activities for the past 5 years since her youngest child graduated from high school. Her daily routine involves cooking for her husband and brother, reading, and watching TV for 6 to 8 hours. She says, "I eat because I have nothing else to do." She is concerned about her eating habits and her recent weight gain.

   a. Using the list of NANDA-approved nursing diagnoses, list several actual and potential (risk) diagnoses for this client. Include a diagnosis related to O.N.'s teaching needs, as learning about diet, blood glucose testing, medication, and activity will contribute to her health and sense of well-being.

      (1) _____

      (2) _____

      (3) _____

      (4) _____

      (5) _____

   Is there a wellness diagnosis that may be appropriate?

   _____

   _____

   b. Now rank your diagnoses according to Maslow's Hierarchy of Needs. Physiological diagnoses have highest priority, followed by safety and security needs and self-esteem.

      (1) _____

      (2) _____

      (3) _____

      (4) _____

      (5) _____

   c. Choose two of your nursing diagnoses for O.N. Write long- and short-term goals and possible interventions.

| Diagnoses | Short-Term Goals—<br>Client will | Long-Term Goals—<br>Client will | Interventions—<br>Nurse will |
|---|---|---|---|
| _____ | (1) _____ | (1) _____ | (1) _____ |
|  | (2) _____ | (2) _____ | (2) _____ |
| _____ | (1) _____ | (1) _____ | (1) _____ |
|  | (2) _____ | (2) _____ | (2) _____ |

6. In what ways is the evaluation phase of the nursing process important to the nurse and the client?

   _____

   _____

a. O.N., your client with diabetes, has returned to your clinic 3 weeks later. How will you deter-mine if O.N. has met her goals?

_____

_____

b. Your assessment indicates that O.N. did not meet a goal of losing weight; in fact, she has gained 2 pounds. In what way will you use this information to reevaluate your goals and interventions?

_____

_____

7. What information could you obtain from documentation tools that could help you provide ap-propriate nursing care for your client?

_____

_____

_____

a. In what ways can accurate and complete documentation help you to communicate informa-tion to other members of the health care team?

_____

_____

b. List three ways documentation helps communication in the health care setting.

   (1) _____

   (2) _____

   (3) _____

c. List two ways documentation supports nursing/health education.

   (1) _____

   (2) _____

d. How does documentation support nursing/health care research?

_____

_____

e. How can documentation help or hurt the nurse in legal situations?

_____

_____

8. On October 12 of this year, you are caring for a 42-year-old female client who is recovering from abdominal surgery. You are now responsible for documentation of her care.

a. Using the sample flowsheet, enter the following information using military time for entries.

Your nursing care included assisting the client with a bed bath and perineal care, but she was able to brush her teeth. You note that she took less than half of her clear liquid diet this morn-ing. Her vital signs at 7:30 A.M. were a temperature of 97.4°F, a pulse of 88, a respiratory rate of 14, and a blood pressure of 128/84.

By the end of your shift, you have noted that her fluid intake included 225 cc po at 8:30 A.M., 50 cc at 11 A.M., and another 320 cc at 1 P.M. She is also receiving IV fluids; by 11 A.M. she had received approximately 500 cc, and another 450 cc by 3 P.M. You emptied her Foley catheter bag for urine twice on your shift; at 11 A.M. there were 350 cc of urine, and at 3 P.M., another 425 cc. She became nauseated and had an emesis of approximately 75 cc after breakfast.

b.  Now document in the Nurse's Progress Record (nurse's notes) the following information on your client.

At 9:15 in the morning, your client said she felt uncomfortable because of a sharp, burning sensation at her surgical incision site. You check her MAR and decide to administer Demerol 50 mg by intramuscular (IM) injection. Thirty minutes later, she tells you she is feeling less pain but is now feeling a little nauseous.

**Nurse's Progress Record**

| Date | Hour | Progress Notes |
|------|------|----------------|
|      |      |                |

*Courtesy of Delmar Cengage Learning*

c.  After writing the entry, you realize you actually gave Demerol 75 mg IM. Now go back to your previous nursing note and correct it appropriately.

d.  You realize at the end of your shift that you forgot to document that your client also complained of a mild headache with her nausea in the morning. What can you do to include it in your notes?

e.  After medicating your client, you realize that Demerol was not the pain medication ordered for your client. Because this is a medication error, what action/documentation should occur?

f.  If you are the nurse responsible for completing the incident report, what information will you include? And who should be notified?

Date:

| Nutrition: | | Hygiene: | | 7-3 | | | 3-11 | | | 11-7 | | |
|---|---|---|---|---|---|---|---|---|---|---|---|---|
| Diet ☐ | NPO ☐ | Bath ☐ Sitz ☐ | | self ☐ assist ☐ total | | | self ☐ assist ☐ total | | | self ☐ assist ☐ total | | |
| Hyperal ☐ Tube Fed ☐ | | Shower ☐ | | refused ☐ ☐ | | | refused ☐ ☐ | | | refused ☐ ☐ | | |
| **Breakfast:** | | Oral Care | | self ☐ | assist ☐ | total ☐ | self ☐ | assist ☐ | total ☐ | self ☐ | assist ☐ | total ☐ |
| All >$\frac{1}{2}$ <$\frac{1}{2}$ 0 | | Shave | | self ☐ | assist ☐ | total ☐ | self ☐ | assist ☐ | total ☐ | self ☐ | assist ☐ | total ☐ |
| ☐ ☐ ☐ ☐ | | Peri Care | | self ☐ | assist ☐ | total ☐ | self ☐ | assist ☐ | total ☐ | self ☐ | assist ☐ | total ☐ |
| **Lunch:** | | Other: | | | | | | | | | | |
| All >$\frac{1}{2}$ <$\frac{1}{2}$ 0 | | Comments: | | | | | | | | | | |
| ☐ ☐ ☐ ☐ | | | | | | | | | | | | |
| **Dinner:** | | | | | | | | | | | | |
| All >$\frac{1}{2}$ <$\frac{1}{2}$ 0 | | | | | | | | | | | | |
| ☐ ☐ ☐ ☐ | | | | | | | | | | | | |
| **Snacks:** | | | | | | | | | | | | |
| All >$\frac{1}{2}$ <$\frac{1}{2}$ 0 | | | | | | | | | | | | |
| ☐ ☐ ☐ ☐ | | | | | | | | | | | | |

| Tube Feeding Residuals | | Intake | | | | | | Output | | | |
|---|---|---|---|---|---|---|---|---|---|---|---|
| Time | Amount | 7-3 | PO | IV | NG & Flush | Enteral | Other | Urine | Ng/Emesis | Stool | Drains |
| | | | | | | | | | | | |
| | | | | | | | | | | | |
| | | | | | | | | | | | |
| | | | | | | | | | | | |
| | | | | | | | | | | | |
| | | 7-3 Total | | | | | | | | | |
| Weight | | 3-11 | | | | | | | | | |
| Today: | | | | | | | | | | | |
| Previous: | | | | | | | | | | | |
| Vital/Signs | | | | | | | | | | | |
| Time | T | P | R | B/P | 3-11 Total | | | | | | |
| | | | | | 11-7 | | | | | | |
| | | | | | | | | | | | |
| | | | | | | | | | | | |
| | | | | | | | | | | | |
| | | | | | 11-7 Total | | | | | | |
| | | | | | 24° Total | | | | | | |

SPOHN HEALTH SYSTEM
SPOHN HOSPITAL
CORPUS CHRISTI, TEXAS 78404

FLOW SHEET—24 HOUR RECORD
PATIENT CARE SERVICES

2705066

NEW: 07/94
REV: 06/26/98
.FM2

4010

*Courtesy of Spohn Health System, Corpus Christi, TX*

## Self-Assessment Questions

Circle the letter that corresponds to the best answer.

1. The primary source of data for the nursing assessment is
   a. the client.
   b. the health history.
   c. nursing observations.
   d. the medical/health record.

2. Which finding is an example of subjective data?
   a. Pain
   b. Weight loss
   c. Diarrhea
   d. Frequency of urination

3. Analysis and synthesis of data occur in which phase of the nursing process?
   a. Planning and outcome identification
   b. Assessment
   c. Evaluation
   d. Diagnosis

4. The nurse determines the priority of the patient diagnoses in the
   a. assessment phase.
   b. diagnosis phase.
   c. planning and outcome identification phase.
   d. evaluation phase.

5. Which statement best describes a primary function of the nursing process?
   a. The nursing process can evaluate and predict patient outcomes.
   b. The nursing process is an organized method of planning and delivering health care.
   c. The nursing process helps the nurse to prioritize care for multiple patient tasks.
   d. The nursing process helps to develop critical-thinking, problem-solving, and decision-making skills.

6. A student shows understanding of the importance of documentation by stating:
   a. "I will avoid using abbreviations to eliminate any confusion."
   b. "I need to be timely and accurate when I write."
   c. "I can save time by telling the next nurse what I did instead of writing it."
   d. "Taking care of the clients is more important than documenting it."

7. Your client has an adverse response to a medication that was ordered for him. You would document this outcome in the
   a. nurse's progress notes.
   b. medication administration record.
   c. incident report.
   d. nursing plan of care.

8. The primary advantage that computerized documentation systems have over written methods is that they
   a. cost less than paper systems.
   b. decrease documentation time.
   c. protect patient confidentiality.
   d. allow alteration of documentation errors.

9. Which of the following statements regarding incident or occurrence reports is incorrect?
   a. Incident reports are most frequently filed due to client falls.
   b. Incident reports are filed to protect the client.
   c. An incident report can alert the facility's insurance company to a possible claim.
   d. When an incident report is filed, it should be documented in the nurse's notes.

10. Oral reporting is most effective when it
   a. includes all laboratory results.
   b. summarizes the entire care of the client.
   c. is structured and organized.
   d. takes place at the bedside.

# Life Span Development

## Key Terms

Match the following terms with their correct definitions.

___ 1. Accommodation

___ 2. Adaptation

___ 3. Adolescence

___ 4. Assimilation

___ 5. Bonding

___ 6. Critical period

___ 7. Development

___ 8. Developmental tasks

___ 9. Embryonic phase

___10. Fetal phase

___11. Germinal phase

___12. Growth

___13. Infancy

___14. Learning

___15. Maturation

a. Onset of the first menstrual period.

b. Component of cognitive development that allows for readjustment of the cognitive structure (mindset) in order to take in new information.

c. Component of cognitive development that involves taking in new experiences or information.

d. Developmental stage that occurs during the first 2 to 8 weeks after fertilization of a human egg.

e. Developmental stage from the ages of 21 years through approximately 40 years.

f. Developmental stage from the ages of 3 years to 6 years.

g. Developmental stage from the ages of 40 years to 65 years.

h. Component of cognitive development that refers to the changes that occur as a result of assimilation and accommodation.

i. Time of the most rapid growth or development in a particular stage of the life cycle during which an individual is most vulnerable to stressors of any type.

j. Developmental stage from the end of the first month to the end of the first year of life.

k. Developmental stage beginning at approximately 12 to 18 months of age, when a child begins to walk, and ending at approximately age 3 years.

l. Individual's perception of self; includes self-esteem, body image, and ideal self.

m. Ability to decide for oneself what is "right."

n. Certain goals that must be achieved during each developmental stage of the life cycle.

o. Developmental stage that begins with conception and lasts approximately 10 to 14 days.

____16. Menarche

____17. Middle adulthood

____18. Moral maturity

____19. Neonatal stage

____20. Older adulthood

____21. Polypharmacy

____22. Preadolescence

____23. Prenatal stage

____24. Preschool stage

____25. Puberty

____26. School-age stage

____27. Self-concept

____28. Sexuality

____29. Spirituality

____30. Teratogenic substance

____31. Toddler stage

____32. Young adulthood

p. First 28 days of life following birth.

q. Developmental stage beginning with conception and ending with birth.

r. Quantitative (measurable) changes in the physical size of the body and its parts.

s. Developmental stage from the ages of approximately 10 years to 12 years.

t. Emergence of secondary sex characteristics that signals the beginning of adolescence.

u. Relationships with one's self, with others, and with a higher power or divine source.

v. Developmental stage from the ages of 12 years to 20 years that begins with the appearance of the secondary sex characteristics (puberty).

w. Developmental stage from the ages of 6 years to 10 years.

x. Behavioral changes in functional abilities and skills.

y. Intrauterine developmental period from 8 weeks to birth.

z. Process of becoming fully grown and developed; involves physiological and behavioral aspects.

aa. Formation of attachment between parent and child; begins at birth when neonate and parents make eye contact.

bb. Process of assimilating information, resulting in a change in behavior.

cc. Substance that can cross the placental barrier and impair normal growth and development.

dd. Developmental stage occurring from the age of 65 years until death.

ee. Recognition of or emphasis on sexual matters.

ff. The use of multiple drugs to treat singular conditions.

## Abbreviation Review

Write the meaning or definition of the following abbreviations, acronyms, and symbols.

1. AIDS _____

2. BSE _____

3. CDC _____

4. CNS _____

5. FAS _____

6. PKU _____

7. STD _____

8. Td _____

9. TSE _____

## Exercises and Activities

1. What is the difference between growth and development?

   _____

   _____

   _____

   a. How do each of the following factors influence growth and development?

   Heredity: _____

   _____

   Life experiences: _____

   _____

   Health status: _____

   _____

   Cultural expectations: _____

   _____

   b. Why is it important for the nurse to understand principles of growth and development?

   _____

   _____

2. According to the following theorists, at what stage would you find each of these individuals?

| Age | Freud | Erikson | Piaget | Sullivan |
|-----|-------|---------|--------|----------|
| Infant | | | | |
| Toddler, age 2 | | | | |
| Adolescent, age 12 | | | | |
| Adult, age 40 | | | | |

   a. What is your own developmental stage according to Erikson's stages of psychosocial development? Why did you select that stage?

   _____

   _____

   Describe yourself in terms of the task to be achieved.

   _____

   _____

   b. What is your stage of cognitive development according to Piaget?

   _____

   _____

How are you achieving the tasks for this stage?

_____

_____

3. Using the diagram, fill in at least one characteristic for each dimension of development (physiological, spiritual, moral, cognitive, psychosocial) for each individual.

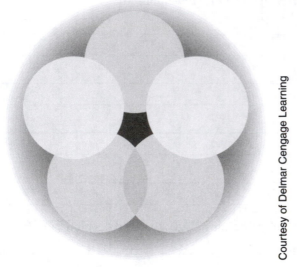

Courtesy of Delmar Cengage Learning

Preschooler, age 4                                     Young adult, age 21

List three nursing implications for each individual:

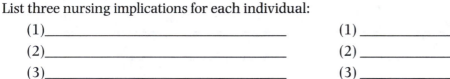

(1)_____          (1) _____

(2)_____          (2) _____

(3)_____          (3) _____

4. List two safety issues for each of the following age groups. Describe two interventions that you could discuss with parents.

| Age Group | Safety Issues | | Interventions | |
|---|---|---|---|---|
| Newborn (first 4 weeks) | 1. | | 1. | |
| | 2. | | 2. | |
| Infant (1 month to 1 year) | 1. | | 1. | |
| | 2. | | 2. | |
| Toddler (12 months to 3 years) | 1. | | 1. | |
| | 2. | | 2. | |
| Preschool (3–6 years) | 1. | | 1. | |
| | 2. | | 2. | |
| School-age child (6–10 years) | 1. | | 1. | |
| | 2. | | 2. | |
| Preadolescence (10–12 years) | 1. | | 1. | |
| | 2. | | 2. | |

5. Respond to the following scenarios.

   a. A.M. is a 16-year-old client who is being seen in the clinic for a sports physical examination. A.M.'s mother, however, expresses concern about her daughter's weight loss over the past several weeks and a change in eating patterns. A.M.'s height and weight are below normal for her age.

   What physiological and psychosocial changes might be particularly important for A.M.?

   _____

   _____

   _____

   _____

   If A.M. were to become your client in a hospital setting, what nursing implications would be important to consider in planning her care?

   _____

   _____

   How can you develop a trusting relationship with A.M.?

   _____

   _____

   What can you do to promote wellness with your adolescent client?

   _____

   _____

   b. T.O., a 2½-year-old child, was brought to the clinic for an immunization. His mother mentions to you that T.O. "still isn't toilet trained" and has become "really picky about what he'll eat." She is worried that he is not getting enough protein and vitamins now.

   Using your knowledge of growth and development for a toddler, how would you address his mother's concerns?

   _____

   _____

   What are the nursing implications for a toddler who is hospitalized?

   _____

   _____

   Why should wellness promotion begin in the early years?

   _____

   _____

6. L.C., a 53-year-old construction worker, comes to the clinic for a routine physical. What physiological changes occur during middle adulthood?

   _____

   _____

   _____

a. Why is maintaining physical activity important for L.C. at this point in his life?

_____

_____

b. It has been seven years since L.C.'s last tetanus shot. L.C. wonders if he should get another one since he is here. How should the nurse reply?

_____

_____

c. He also wonders about receiving a flu vaccination. How should the nurse respond?

_____

_____

d. What safety concerns should the nurse address with L.C. since he is middle-aged?

_____

_____

## Self-Assessment Questions

Circle the letter that corresponds to the best answer.

1. The principles of growth and development include all but which of the following?
   a. Some stages are more critical than others.
   b. Development occurs in a head-to-toe direction.
   c. The pattern is continuous, orderly, and predictable.
   d. Development occurs in a distal to proximal manner.

2. An individual's ability to adapt effectively to stressors results primarily from
   a. life experiences.
   b. hereditary factors.
   c. a positive self-concept.
   d. moral maturity and spirituality.

3. The nurse encourages early and frequent parent–infant interaction to facilitate
   a. parenting skills.
   b. bonding and trust.
   c. anticipatory guidance.
   d. cognitive development.

4. The nurse caring for a toddler understands that the greatest source of stress in the hospital relates to the
   a. separation from the parents.
   b. lack of familiar surroundings.
   c. symptoms of the illness or injury.
   d. anxiety over medical procedures.

5. The nurse anticipating a teaching procedure for a 60-year-old client would include health screening recommendations, exercise and weight control, and
   a. coping with loss.
   b. suicide prevention.
   c. acceptance of aging.
   d. time management skills.

6. A 5-year-old child would be in Erikson's stage of
   a. autonomy vs. shame and doubt.
   b. initiative vs. guilt.
   c. industry vs. inferiority.
   d. identity vs. role confusion.

7. Which of these methods for bottle-feeding should *not* be avoided?
   a. Using the bottle as a pacifier
   b. Using the microwave to heat bottles
   c. Propping the bottle for feeding
   d. Placing the baby in a semireclining position

8. The nurse would teach a toddler's parent that
   a. using food as a reward is beneficial.
   b. serving large portions will ensure that the toddler eats.
   c. the toddler may have sporadic eating patterns.
   d. snacks are not necessary to meet dietary requirements.

9. In preadolescent boys, the first signs of puberty include
   a. testicular enlargement.
   b. pubic hair growth.
   c. thickening of the scrotum.
   d. both a. and b.

10. While assessing an adolescent, a nurse notices a neglect of personal hygiene and loss of interest in pleasurable activities. These can be signs of
    a. suicide risk.
    b. pain.
    c. rebelling.
    d. impulsive behavior.

# Cultural Considerations

## Key Terms

Match the following terms with their correct definitions.

____ 1. Acculturation

____ 2. Agnostic

____ 3. Atheist

____ 4. Cultural assimilation

____ 5. Cultural diversity

____ 6. Culture

____ 7. Dominant culture

____ 8. Ethnicity

____ 9. Ethnocentrism

____10. Minority group

____11. Oppression

____12. Race

____13. Religious support system

a. Opposing forces that, when in balance, yield health.

b. Group of ministers, priests, rabbis, nuns, or laypersons who are able to meet clients' spiritual needs in the health care setting.

c. Cultural group's perception of itself or a group identity.

d. Process of learning norms, beliefs, and behavioral expectations of a group.

e. Process whereby individuals from a minority group are absorbed by the dominant culture and take on the characteristics of the dominant culture.

f. Dynamic and integrated structures of knowledge, beliefs, behaviors, ideas, attitudes, values, habits, customs, languages, symbols, rituals, ceremonies, and practices that are unique to a particular group of people.

g. Assumption of cultural superiority and an inability to accept other cultures' ways of organizing reality.

h. Condition wherein the rules, modes, and ideals of one group are imposed on another group.

i. Recognition of spiritual needs and the assistance given toward meeting those needs.

j. Individual who believes that the existence of God cannot be proved or disproved.

k. Differences among people that result from racial, ethnic, and cultural variables.

l. Group of people who constitute less than a numerical majority of the population and who, because of their cultural, racial, ethnic, religious, or other characteristics, are often labeled and treated differently from others in the society.

m. Individual's desire to find meaning and purpose in life, pain, and death.

____14. Spiritual care

____15. Spiritual needs

____16. Stereotyping

____17. Yin and yang

n. Individual who does not believe in God or any other deity.

o. Group whose values prevail within a society.

p. Grouping of people based on biological similarities such as physical characteristics.

q. Belief that all people within the same racial, ethnic, or cultural group act alike and share the same beliefs and attitudes.

## Abbreviation Review

Write the meaning or definition of the following abbreviations.

1. WASP _____

2. WHO _____

## Exercises and Activities

1. How do the terms *ethnicity* and *race* differ in meaning?

   _____

   _____

   _____

   a. How would you explain the term *cultural diversity* to another student?

   _____

   _____

   b. In what ways does cultural diversity of health care workers, clients, and community populations affect you and your clients in today's health care settings?

   _____

   _____

2. Describe your own cultural background using the Cultural Assessment Guide.

   _____

   _____

   _____

   _____

   _____

   _____

## CULTURAL ASSESSMENT GUIDE

Name _____

Other names or nicknames _____

Date of birth _____ Place of birth _____

Primary language _____ Other languages _____

Religious affiliation _____

Describe how you identify with your cultural group. _____

Define your ethnic group. _____

Describe your beliefs or customs about:

    Life _____

    Health _____

    Illness _____

    Death _____

How do you best learn? Seeing (Visual) _____ Hearing (Auditory) _____
Doing (Kinesthetic) _____

What foods are forbidden by your religion or culture? _____
_____

What are your food preferences? _____

Give examples of your family's dietary habits. _____
_____

How do your religious practices and beliefs affect your life when in good health? _____
_____

When in poor health? _____

Who provides your health care services? _____
_____

What cultural health practices are you aware of, and which do you utilize? _____
_____

List cultural restrictions that your caregiver needs to know. _____
_____

Describe how your family members relate to and communicate with each other. _____
_____

What or who is your primary source of health information? _____
_____

What other cultural beliefs would you like to share? _____
_____

a. Choose two cultural groups different from your own. Compare and contrast your beliefs/customs concerning each of the following topics with what you know about those beliefs/customs of the other cultural groups.

| *Your Beliefs/Customs* | *Cultural Group:*_____ | *Cultural Group:*_____ |
|---|---|---|
| Family structure | | |
| Time orientation | | |
| Religion | | |
| What causes disease | | |
| Who provides health care | | |
| Special healing practices | | |

b. How might each of the following affect health care practices?

Religious beliefs: _____

_____

Family structure: _____

_____

Time orientation: _____

_____

Nutritional preferences: _____

_____

3. In which cultural or religious group would you find each of the following beliefs or health practices?

_____ Cupping may be used to draw out evil or illness.

_____ A talisman worn around the wrist or neck wards off disease.

_____ A healing ritual called the Blessingway ceremony may be performed.

_____ Traditional healers include the *curandero* and *yerbero*.

_____ Prayers to Allah may be offered five times a day.

_____ Traditional healers include the shaman.

_____ Illness can be eliminated through prayer and spiritual understanding.

_____ Male circumcision is a religious custom performed 8 days after birth.

_____ Blood and blood products are usually refused.

_____ A special undergarment may be worn that symbolizes dedication to God.

a. Describe how you might feel about caring for each of the following clients.

A client who relies on folk remedies and healers: _____

_____

A client who responds to pain in a different way than you: _____

_____

A client who is using healing rituals and ceremonies: _____

_____

b.  In what ways does each of the following religions support the spiritual needs of an ill client?

Christian Science: _____

_____

Judaism: _____

_____

Islam: _____

_____

Protestantism: _____

_____

Roman Catholicism: _____

_____

4.  You are assigned to care for Y.H., a 68-year-old client who has been admitted to your hospital for congestive heart failure. She and her husband have been in the United States for 2 months to visit their son and had planned on returning home before Y.H. became ill. As you enter her room to do a physical assessment, you note that she is wearing traditional clothing with only her face and hands exposed, rather than her hospital gown. Her husband, who speaks limited English, sits next to her. Y.H. appears anxious and uncomfortable but doesn't respond to your questions about pain. You want to help your client but are unfamiliar with her culture and religion.

a.  In what ways can health care givers support Y.H.'s religious beliefs while she is hospitalized?

_____

_____

b.  List two nursing diagnoses with cultural implications that might be appropriate for your client.

(1) _____

(2) _____

c.  How can members of Y.H.'s family assist you in providing culturally sensitive nursing care?

_____

_____

d.  If you are caring for a client of a cultural or religious group with which you are unfamiliar, how could you determine the special needs/support for your client?

_____

_____

e.  Y.H. speaks very little English. How does the nurse explain care and treatment to Y.H.?

_____

_____

f.  Y.H. family wishes to bring her food from home. She is on a general diet. How should the nurse respond to the request?

_____

_____

5. Nurses are expected to deliver culturally competent care. What does this statement mean?

   _____

   _____

   _____

6. The nurse cares for a new refugee from Haiti. The client smiles and nods her head as if she is in agreement with the plan of care. How does the nurse validate that the client understands the treatments?

   _____

   _____

   _____

   a. The client clutches an amulet tightly while the nurse is in the room. How should the nurse respond to this foreign object?

      _____

      _____

7. The nurse admitting M.K. to the unit for leukemia notes that M.K. is of the Jehovah's Witness faith. Explain how the usual treatment plan may have to be altered to accommodate M.K.'s faith.

   _____

   _____

   _____

   a. What dietary accommodations should the nurse consider for M.K.?

      _____

      _____

8. J.B., an elderly Roman Catholic male patient, has pneumonia and is very ill. The priest visiting with him asks if J.B. may receive communion. How should the nurse respond?

   _____

   _____

   a. J.B.'s family asks for "last rites." Explain what this means.

      _____

      _____

   b. What should the nurse do if presented with the request for the Sacrement of the Sick?

      _____

      _____

# Self-Assessment Questions

Circle the letter that corresponds to the best answer.

1. The first priority for the nurse providing culturally sensitive care is to
   a. accommodate differences when possible.
   b. identify the client's cultural/religious group.
   c. examine one's own cultural and personal beliefs.
   d. listen for cues in the client's conversation about ethnic beliefs.

2. A time orientation to the past may be demonstrated by which of the following cultural groups?
   a. Asian American
   b. Native American
   c. African American
   d. Hispanic American

3. The process of learning the norms, beliefs, and behaviors of a culture is referred to as
   a. ethnocentrism.
   b. cultural assimilation.
   c. socialization.
   d. acculturation.

4. The nurse is caring for an Asian American client who refuses ice water and the cold foods served for her meal. The nurse recognizes that because of the client's cultural background, her refusal is most likely due to her
   a. acceptance of a supernatural cause for disease.
   b. belief in a yin and yang etiology of disease.
   c. preference for her own family's foods.
   d. attempt to cleanse her body of unhealthy organisms.

5. Which of the following statements is true concerning cultural influence on health care?
   a. All cultures value health and good medical practice.
   b. Response to health and illness varies according to cultural origin.
   c. Knowing a client's cultural identity allows the nurse to make certain assumptions.
   d. Clients from all cultures respond positively to the nurse's caring touch.

6. An area not affected by culture is
   a. attitude.
   b. beliefs.
   c. values.
   d. All are affected by culture.

7. Labeling people according to cultural preconceptions is called
   a. oppression.
   b. stereotyping.
   c. cultural characteristics.
   d. ethnocentrism.

8. An inability to accept another culture's ways is called
   a. oppression.
   b. stereotyping.
   c. cultural characteristics.
   d. ethnocentrism.

9. Which statement is *not* an identified cultural characteristic?
   a. Culture is learned.
   b. Culture is integrated.
   c. Culture is inherited.
   d. Culture is dynamic.

10. Agnostics believe
    a. that the existence of God cannot be proved or disproved.
    b. that God does not exist.
    c. that a believer will reach an age of understanding.
    d. in reincarnation.

# Stress, Adaptation, and Anxiety

## Key Terms

Match the following terms with their correct definitions.

___ 1. Adaptation

___ 2. Adaptive energy

___ 3. Adaptive measure

___ 4. Anxiety

___ 5. Burnout

___ 6. Catharsis

___ 7. Change

___ 8. Change agent

___ 9. Conditioning

___10. Cognitive reframing

___11. Crisis

___12. Crisis intervention

___13. Defense mechanism

___14. Depersonalization

___15. Distress

a. State of physical and emotional exhaustion that occurs when caregivers deplete their adaptive energy.

b. Ongoing process whereby individuals use various responses to adjust to stressors and change.

c. Person who intentionally creates and implements change.

d. Measure used to avoid conflict or stress.

e. Teaching a person a behavior until it becomes an automatic response; method of conserving adaptive energy.

f. Inner forces that an individual uses to adapt to stress (phrase coined by Selye).

g. Stress that results in positive outcomes.

h. Any situation, event, or agent that produces stress.

i. Physiological response to a stressor (e.g., trauma, illness) affecting a specific part of the body.

j. Acute state of disorganization that occurs when the individual's usual coping mechanisms are no longer effective.

k. Measure for coping with stress that requires a minimal amount of energy.

l. Specific technique used to assist clients in regaining equilibrium.

m. State wherein the body becomes physiologically ready to defend itself by either fighting or running away from the danger.

n. Nonspecific response to any demand made on the body (Selye, 1974).

o. Subjective response that occurs when a person experiences a real or a perceived threat to well-being; a diverse feeling of dread or apprehension.

___16. Endorphins

p. Process of talking out one's feelings; "getting things off the chest" through verbalization.

___17. Eustress

q. Unconscious operation that protects the mind from anxiety.

___18. Fight-or-flight response

r. Dynamic process whereby an individual's response to a stressor leads to an alteration in behavior.

___19. General adaptation syndrome

s. Subjective experience that occurs when stressors evoke an ineffective response.

___20. Homeostasis

t. Physiological response that occurs when a person experiences a stressor.

___21. Local adaptation syndrome

u. Treating an individual as an object rather than as a person.

___22. Maladaptive measure

v. Balance or equilibrium among the physiological, psychological, sociocultural, intellectual, and spiritual needs of the body.

___23. Stress

w. Group of opiate-like substances produced naturally by the brain, which raise the pain threshold, produce sedation and euphoria, and promote a sense of well-being.

___24. Stressor

x. Stress-management technique whereby the individual changes a negative perception of a situation or event to a more positive, less threatening perception.

## Abbreviation Review

Write the meaning or definition of the following abbreviations and acronyms.

1. CVA _____

2. GAS _____

3. LAS _____

4. NANDA _____

## Exercises and Activities

1. Differentiate stress and anxiety.

_____

_____

_____

a. How are low levels of anxiety helpful to an individual?

_____

_____

b. What can happen when stress intensifies or continues for a long period?

_____

_____

c. What role does client education play in helping to manage stress?

_____

_____

d. Why are a healthy diet and physical exercise valuable for stress management?

_____

_____

2. Think of a stressful event that has occurred in your life. Briefly describe the event or situation that was a source of stress.

_____

_____

_____

a. What manifestations of stress did you experience (physiological, psychological, cognitive, behavioral, and spiritual)?

_____

_____

b. What coping mechanisms did you use?

_____

_____

c. If a similar situation would occur in the future, in what ways might you respond differently?

_____

_____

3. A nurse is working the night shift in a busy unit at a large tertiary care center. Her nursing responsibilities, which once seemed like a challenge, are now overwhelming. Clients are sicker; it seems like there is a constant staff shortage; and once again, the unit will have a new nurse manager. The nurse volunteered to work on two important nursing committees and has often adjusted her schedule to accommodate other staff members' needs. She thought working the night shift would give her more time with her family, but she has never adapted to sleeping during the day and seldom feels well rested. With two teenagers and a 9-year-old at home, there never seem to be enough hours in the day. She is becoming short-tempered at work and at home.

a. How does stress contribute to burnout in the nursing profession?

_____

_____

b. What are the stressors in the nurse's life?

_____

_____

c. Suggest two strategies that she could use at work to help her cope.

_____

_____

d. What would you recommend to this nurse to help her manage stress in her life?

_____

_____

4. C.G. is a 31-year-old father of two children, ages 8 and 5, and has been enjoying a successful career working for a construction company. He has recently been diagnosed with multiple sclerosis following progressive muscle weakness and now also with some problems with a visual disturbance. In addition to his medical bills and physical needs, he is worried about his job and the ability of his wife to handle additional responsibilities at home.

   a. Write two nursing diagnoses for C.G.

   (1) _____

   (2) _____

   b. C.G. may experience long-term stress related to his illness and possible job loss. In what ways might this affect his illness or adaptation?

   _____

   _____

   c. What specific suggestions could you make to help C.G.?

   _____

   _____

   d. Why would it be important to involve family members in this situation?

   _____

   _____

5. Explain how a person who is healthy demonstrates adaptation.

   _____

   _____

   _____

6. What are the characteristcs of a crisis?

   _____

   _____

   _____

   a. Explain how a crisis is *not* mental illness.

   _____

   _____

7. Describe how a nurse might be a change agent.

   _____

   _____

   _____

8. Identify three traits necessary for a nurse to adapt to change.

   (1) _____

   (2) _____

   (3) _____

9. The owner of a small business is in the hosipital on bedrest with a fractured leg. He tripped over an electric cord at work. As the nurse is providing care to him, he admits that he is worried about how his business is operating without him. He is concerned that OSHA will investigate his fall and whether his insurance will cover the cost of his hospitalization. Additionally, his wife just lost her job at a local factory, and his 16-year-old daughter wants to get married and move out of the house. The nurse recognizes that he needs to verbalize his feelings. What are the effects of verbalization?

   _____

   _____

   _____

   a. The nurse recognizes that the client needs less stress and external stimuli. How can this be accomplished?

   _____

   _____

   b. What are some stress management techniques that the nurse can use with this client?

   _____

   _____

## Self-Assessment Questions

Circle the letter that corresponds to the best answer.

1. A client with chronic obstructive pulmonary disease who continues to smoke may be exhibiting a defense mechanism called
   a. denial.
   b. avoidance.
   c. suppression.
   d. rationalization.

2. An individual's ability to use problem-solving skills to cope with stress or change is
   a. behavioral change.
   b. cognitive reframing.
   c. cognitive adaptation.
   d. psychological adaptation.

3. An individual's response to stressors, according to the general adaptation syndrome, occurs in three stages, which include alarm, resistance, and
   a. exhaustion.
   b. adaptation.
   c. homeostasis.
   d. fight-or-flight response.

4. Your client appears tense and is complaining of headache and nausea. Because your client has been dealing with a stressful situation for some time, you realize that these may be symptoms of
   a. mild anxiety.
   b. moderate anxiety.
   c. severe anxiety.
   d. denial.

5. A primary nursing intervention for the client experiencing mild anxiety is to
   a. provide limits and structure.
   b. develop appropriate diagnoses.
   c. minimize environmental stimuli.
   d. use the opportunity for teaching.

6. The nurse caring for a client who is experiencing panic should first
   a. encourage catharsis.
   b. maintain client safety.
   c. teach coping methods.
   d. focus the client on specific tasks.

7. Which statement is *not* an aspect of a stressor?
   a. A stressor is neutral.
   b. A pleasant event cannot be a stressor.
   c. The individual's perception of a stressor will determine its effect.
   d. A stressor can be internal or external.

8. Physiological effects that occur in the first stage of GAS are
   a. relaxation of respiratory muscles, maintenance of blood pressure, and slowing of the digestive system.
   b. inflammatory suppression, dilated pupils, and exhaustion.
   c. fluid retention, gluconeogenesis, and increased energy.
   d. epinephrine secretion, decrease in heart rate, and fatigue.

9. Physiological effects that occur in the second stage of GAS are
   a. relaxation of respiratory muscles, maintenance of blood pressure, and slowing of the digestive system.
   b. inflammatory suppression, dilated pupils, and exhaustion.
   c. fluid retention, gluconeogenesis, and increased energy.
   d. epinephrine secretion, decrease in heart rate, and fatigue.

10. Outcomes of stress include
    a. personal growth.
    b. disorganization.
    c. distress.
    d. All can be outcomes of stress.

# End-of-Life Care

## Key Terms

Match the following terms with their correct definitions.

| | |
|---|---|
| ___ 1. Advance directive | a. Breathing characterized by periods of apnea alternating with periods of dyspnea. |
| ___ 2. Algor mortis | b. Persistent pattern of intense grief that does not result in reconciliation of feelings. |
| ___ 3. Anticipatory grief | c. Imagining the feeling of horror felt by a victim or reliving the terror of an incident. |
| ___ 4. Autopsy | d. Form of reminiscence wherein a client attempts either to come to terms with conflict or to gain meaning from life and die peacefully. |
| ___ 5. Bereavement | e. Loss that occurs as a result of moving from one developmental stage to another. |
| ___ 6. Breakthrough pain | f. Period of grief following the death of a loved one. |
| ___ 7. Cheyne-Stokes respirations | g. Care given immediately after death before the body is moved to the mortuary. |
| ___ 8. Complicated grief | h. Covering for the body after death. |
| ___ 9. Death rattle | i. Decrease in body temperature after death, resulting in lack of skin elasticity. |
| ___ 10. Disenfranchised grief | j. Grief associated with traumatic death such as death by homicide, violence, or accident; a survivor suffers emotions of greater intensity than those associated with normal grief. |
| ___ 11. Dysfunctional grief | k. Bluish purple discoloration of the skin, usually at pressure points, that is a by-product of red blood cell destruction. |
| ___ 12. End-of-life care | l. Funeral home. |
| ___ 13. Grief | m. Occurrence of grief work before an expected loss actually occurs. |
| ___ 14. Health Care Surrogate Law | n. Care that relieves symptoms, such as pain, but does not alter the course of disease. |

___15. Hospice

o. Stiffening of the body that occurs 2 to 4 hours after death as a result of contraction of skeletal and smooth muscles.

___16. Life review

p. Sudden, acute, temporary pain that is usually precipitated by a treatment, a procedure, or unusual activity of the client.

___17. Liver mortis

q. "Grief that is not openly acknowledged, socially sanctioned, or publicly shared" (Doka, Rushton, & Thorstenson, 1994).

___18. Loss

r. Law enacted by some states that provides a legal means for decision making in the absence of advance directives.

___19. Maturational loss

s. Support measures implemented to restore consciousness and life.

___20. Mortuary

t. Grief reaction that normally follows a significant loss.

___21. Mourning

u. Any situation, either actual, potential, or perceived, wherein a valued object or person is changed or is no longer accessible to the individual.

___22. Palliative care

v. Examination of a body after death by a pathologist to determine cause.

___23. Postmortem care

w. Breathing sound in the period preceding death caused by a collection of secretions in the larynx.

___24. Resuscitation

x. Care of the terminally ill founded on the concept of allowing individuals to die with dignity and surrounded by those who love them.

___25. Rigor mortis

y. Loss that occurs in response to external events that are usually beyond the individual's control.

___26. Shroud

z. Period of time during which grief is expressed and resolution and integration of the loss occur.

___27. Situational loss

aa. Series of intense physical and psychological responses that occurs following a loss; a normal, natural, necessary, and adaptive response to a loss.

___28. Traumatic imagery

bb. Nursing care of the terminally ill that focuses on the physical and psychological needs of the patient and family.

___29. Uncomplicated grief

cc. Any written instruction recognized under state law, including a durable power of attorney, for health care or living will.

## Abbreviation Review

Write the meaning or definition of the following abbreviations and acronyms.

1. ANA _____

2. DNR _____

3. HMO _____

4. IM _____

5. MS _____

6. NANDA _____

7. OBRA _____

8. PSDA _____

9. PTSD _____

10. SIDS _____

11. TB _____

## Exercises and Activities

1. Why is mourning an important process for an individual who is experiencing a loss?

   _____

   _____

   _____

   a. Briefly describe each of the following types of loss.

   External object: _____

   Familiar environment: _____

   Aspect of self: _____

   Significant other: _____

   b. Give two examples of loss for each developmental stage.

   Childhood            (1) _____

                        (2) _____

   Adolescence          (1) _____

                        (2) _____

   Early adulthood      (1) _____

                        (2) _____

   Middle adulthood     (1) _____

                        (2) _____

   Late adulthood       (1) _____

                        (2) _____

2. Choose one type of loss that you have experienced. Briefly describe the loss and any feelings of grief that may have accompanied it.

   _____

   _____

   _____

   a. Did your feelings of grief resolve? If so, how long did the process take?

   _____

   _____

   b. What actions or statements by others were most helpful?

   _____

   _____

c. Were any actions or statements not helpful?

_____

_____

3. Differentiate dysfunctional and disenfranchised grief.

_____

_____

_____

a. Why might an abortion cause an individual to experience disenfranchised grief?

_____

_____

b. How might the grief response differ for parents who have lost an infant to sudden infant death syndrome versus a neonatal death for other reasons?

_____

_____

c. Why is the loss of a child considered one of the most difficult?

_____

_____

4. One of your clients today is N.W., a 25-year-old woman who is terminally ill with ovarian cancer, diagnosed shortly after the birth of her second child a few months ago. She completed a round of chemotherapy that was extremely difficult for her and had little effect on the cancer. After much thought, she has made the decision not to continue therapy. Her primary concern now is her husband and the welfare of her children. P.W. appears to be in denial at times, or is angry with her physician for not diagnosing the disease earlier. There are many issues he needs to face, including taking over the care of both children.

a. According to Kübler-Ross's stages of dying and death, what stage do you feel N.W. is in?

_____

What stage is her husband in?

_____

b. How might anticipatory grief be helpful for her husband?

_____

_____

How might it be a disadvantage?

_____

_____

c. N.W. and P.W. have a 4-year-old child at home. How does a child at that age perceive dying?

_____

_____

d. What role could hospice play in helping N.W. and her family cope with her impending death?

_____

_____

e. N.W. and her husband have finally discussed her wishes concerning terminal care. What documents should she complete?

_____

_____

f. List four physiological changes that occur as death becomes imminent, and signs or symptoms that accompany each.

(1) _____

(2) _____

(3) _____

(4) _____

g. You find yourself having difficulty dealing with N.W.'s death, as you had become fond of her and very involved in her care. What symptoms might indicate that you are in need of grief counseling? What actions might be helpful to deal with the loss?

_____

_____

_____

_____

5. G.H. has multiple sclerosis that no longer reponds to treatment. His condition has deteriorated to the piont he is unable to swallow liquids, talk, or care for himself. He will be entering a hospice unit. How are hospice and palliative care different?

_____

_____

_____

a. M.H., his wife, would like to know what the goals of treatment for him are now. How does the nurse explain this to her?

_____

_____

b. M.H. is concerned that G.H. has lost interest in food and drink. How should the nurse explain this?

_____

_____

c. G.H. complains of pain and rates his pain as an 8 out of 10. he has a prescription for morphine liquid 10 mg every 4 hours, but it does not seem to be working. What can the nurse do to increase G.H.'s comfort level?

_____

_____

    d. Explain the World Health Organization's three-step ladder for pain control.

_____

_____

    e. G.H. can hardly speak because of the multiple sclerosis. What nonverbal cues will the nurse observe for when assessing his comfort level?

_____

_____

    f. Why might Fentanyl become the drug of choice for pain managment with G.H.?

_____

_____

    g. M.H. wants to stay with her husband around the clock. She tells the nurse that they have been married for 58 years and have never been apart. How can the nurse accommodate M.H.'s request?

_____

_____

    h. A student nurse has been assigned to care for G.H. today. The nurse asks the student nurse to identify the physical signs of death. How does the student nurse respond?

_____

_____

    i. G.H. finally dies and the nurse notes the time of death. The nurse has explained to the student nurse that the postmortem cares must be completed. What does this mean?

_____

_____

    j. The nurse says she is relieved that G.H.'s suffering is finally over. The student nurse asks the nurse how the nurse handles her emotions. How should the nurse respond to the student?

_____

_____

## Self-Assessment Questions

Circle the letter that corresponds to the best answer.

    1. Your client experienced the death of her spouse several months ago. She continues to talk about him and the death repeatedly and is having difficulty eating and sleeping. This client is experiencing
        a. absent grief.
        b. detachment.
        c. dysfunctional grief.
        d. loss of patterns of conduct.

    2. When dealing with a child who is experiencing the loss of a parent or sibling, the nurse should
        a. avoid using euphemisms like the person is "gone to sleep" in reference to death.
        b. offer thoughtful explanations about abstract ideas like death.
        c. encourage the child to get over the loss as quickly as possible.
        d. protect the child from potentially frightening places like the mortuary.

3. The nurse is caring for a client with terminal cancer. Nursing interventions for this client that focus on relieving symptoms such as pain are called
   a. respite care.
   b. palliative care.
   c. adjuvant therapy.
   d. anticipatory support.

4. The nurse understands that a client with a living will and durable power of attorney
   a. is required to sign the Patient Self-Determination form.
   b. relinquishes the right to make health care decisions.
   c. has a life-threatening disease or terminal illness.
   d. still needs a "do not resuscitate" medical order.

5. According to Kübler-Ross, the fifth and final stage of dying experienced by an individual is
   a. life review.
   b. resignation.
   c. acceptance.
   d. hopefulness.

6. The first stage of grief is
   a. acceptance.
   b. recovery.
   c. shock.
   d. anger.

7. During the second stage of grief, a person may feel
   a. anger and guilt.
   b. emotional numbness.
   c. able to live again.
   d. a positive attitude.

8. The *inability* to conclude grieving is called
   a. masked grief.
   b. exaggerated grief.
   c. delayed grief.
   d. chronic grief.

9. What developmental disruption may occur in a school-age child experiencing the loss of a parent?
   a. Long-lasting psychosocial problems
   b. Belief that death was his/her fault
   c. Potential death-avoidance behavior
   d. Difficulty forming intimate relationships

10. Which type of death with a negative stigma may prohibit survivors from successfully resolving their guilt?
    a. Unexpected death
    b. Suicide
    c. Traumatic death
    d. Neonatal death

# Wellness Concepts

## Key Terms

Match the following terms with their correct definitions.

____ 1. Genogram

____ 2. Health

____ 3. Prevention

____ 4. Primary prevention

____ 5. Secondary prevention

____ 6. Tertiary prevention

____ 7. Wellness

a. Early detection, diagnosis, screening, and intervention, generally before symptoms appear, to reduce the consequences of a health problem.

b. State of optimal health wherein an individual moves toward integration of human functioning, maximizes human potential, takes responsibility for health, and has greater self-awareness and self-satisfaction.

c. According to the World Health Organization, the state of complete physical, mental, and social well-being, not merely the absence of disease or infirmity.

d. Hindering, obstructing, or thwarting a disease or illness.

e. Treatment of an illness or disease after symptoms have appeared so as to prevent further progression.

f. All practices designed to keep health problems from developing.

g. Method of visualizing family members, their birth and death dates or ages, and specific health problems.

## Abbreviation Review

Write the meaning or definition of the following abbreviations and acronyms.

1. AIDS _____

2. BMI _____

3. CDC _____

4. ECG _____

5. EKG _____

6. Hgb _____

7. HIV _____

8. LDL _____

9. Pap _____

10. PHS _____

11. SPF _____

12. USDHHS _____

13. WHO _____

## Exercises and Activities

1. Write your own definition of wellness as you believe it applies to you. Include behaviors in each of the seven areas of wellness: emotional, mental, intellectual, vocational, social, spiritual, and physical.

   _____

   _____

   _____

   _____

   _____

   a. Choose three of the areas of wellness and describe what you could do to promote wellness for yourself in each of those areas.

      (1) _____

      (2) _____

      (3) _____

   b. Describe your concept of wellness as it might apply to an elderly client.

      _____

      _____

2. List three overall goals for the Healthy People 2010 objective.

   a. _____

   b. _____

   c. _____

3. Review Table 14-1 in your text. Look at the objectives for physical activity and fitness, nutrition, and AIDS/HIV infection. Briefly describe each objective and state whether the objective met the year 2000 target. If the target was not met, give a possible reason.

   Physical activity and fitness _____

   _____

   Nutrition _____

   _____

   AIDS/HIV infection _____

   _____

4. In what ways can nurses be involved in helping to achieve the goals of Healthy People 2010?

   _____

   _____

5. Why are preconception and prenatal health important?

_____

_____

_____

6. List the four factors affecting health. Describe the role each factor plays in determining the health of an individual.

a. _____

b. _____

c. _____

d. _____

7. Define each type of prevention and give two examples.

| | Definition | Examples |
|---|---|---|
| Primary | | (1) |
| | | (2) |
| Secondary | | (1) |
| | | (2) |
| Tertiary | | (1) |
| | | (2) |

8. N.T. is a 20-year-old college student who is studying computer programming. Although she finds her courses interesting, she is becoming increasingly stressed about her class load and grades. Struggling to maintain a passing average, she has started smoking again, after quitting 6 months ago. She has regained several pounds that she had previously lost through diet and exercise. To pay for classes, N.T. has been working 25 hours a week at a restaurant. Her boyfriend, with whom she is sexually active, tries to be supportive. Because of her schedule she has little time for exercise, and she knows she shouldn't be smoking but can't stop.

a. What health problems might N.T. encounter if she continues with her present lifestyle?

_____

_____

b. What changes would be most helpful to N.T. at this time?

_____

_____

c. Recommend three methods of stress reduction for N.T.

_____

_____

d. At N.T.'s age, what routine exams would you suggest she have?

_____

_____

e. After reviewing a genogram with information regarding N.T.'s family, you determine that she is also at an increased risk for osteoporosis. What steps could you recommend to N.T. that might prevent or reduce her risk for this disease?

_____

_____

## Self-Assessment Questions

Circle the letter that corresponds to the best answer.

1. Which of the following areas has the most factors affecting health and wellness?
   a. Genetics and human biology
   b. Environmental influences
   c. Personal behavior
   d. Health care

2. Monthly breast self-examination is an example of which of the following?
   a. Primary prevention
   b. Secondary prevention
   c. Tertiary prevention
   d. Early intervention

3. A major goal of Healthy People 2010 is to
   a. increase access to preventive services.
   b. provide more health care workers.
   c. establish health care guidelines.
   d. identify concepts of wellness.

4. An important part of tertiary prevention is
   a. screening.
   b. rehabilitation.
   c. health promotion.
   d. consumer awareness.

5. A client who is experiencing excessive stress is at risk for accidents, heart disease, and
   a. stroke.
   b. cancer.
   c. diabetes.
   d. atherosclerosis.

6. Health care employers are required to provide
   a. child care.
   b. hepatitis B vaccination.
   c. stress reduction.
   d. prophylaxis exams.
7. A genogram should include
   a. one generation.
   b. two generations.
   c. three generations.
   d. four generations.

8. A guideline to promote healthy living for the prevention of heart disease can include
   a. a low-fiber diet.
   b. weekly exercise.
   c. having a physical exam every 5 years.
   d. maintaining an appropriate weight.

9. A guideline to promote healthy living for the prevention of cancer can include
   a. limiting smoking.
   b. a low-fiber diet.
   c. limiting alcohol intake.
   d. going to sun-tanning booths.

10. Wellness encompasses
    a. prevention.
    b. early detection.
    c. treatment of health problems.
    d. All are factors of wellness.

# Self-Concept

## Key Terms

Match the following terms with their correct definitions.

| | | |
|---|---|---|
| ___ 1. Body image | a. | How one really thinks about oneself. |
| ___ 2. Empowerment | b. | What individuals think others think of them. |
| ___ 3. Ideal self | c. | Consciously knowing how the self thinks, feels, believes, and behaves at a specific time. |
| ___ 4. Identity | d. | One's perception of physical self. |
| ___ 5. Public self | e. | A helping process and partnerships through which individuals are enabled to make change. |
| ___ 6. Real self | f. | An individual's perception of self. |
| ___ 7. Role | g. | Specific behaviors that a person exhibits in each role. |
| ___ 8. Role performance | h. | An ascribed or assumed expected behavior in a social situation. |
| ___ 9. Self-awareness | i. | The person that the client would like to be. |
| ___10. Self-concept | j. | One's personal opinion of oneself. |
| ___11. Self-esteem | k. | An individual's conscious description of who he or she is. |

## Abbreviation Review

Write the meaning or definition of the following abbreviations, acronyms, and symbols.

1. NANDA _____

## Exercises and Activities

1. What are some characteristics of clients with positive self-concepts?

   _____

   _____

   _____

2. Using the memory trick **I LIKE ME**, identify nursing interventions used to promote a positive self-concept.

I _____

L _____

I _____

K _____

E _____

M _____

E _____

3. Discuss how health-related factors may affect body image.

_____

_____

_____

4. How might nurses teach clients to increase their self-image?

_____

_____

_____

5. Explain how an individual's self-concept develops across the life span.

Infancy _____

Childhood _____

Adolescence _____

Adulthood _____

## Self-Assessment Questions

Circle the letter that corresponds to the best answer.

1. The nurse assesses the client's vital signs and gathers data about the client's health history and psychological factors such as spirituality. These specific behaviors are known as
   a. role performance.
   b. real self.
   c. public self.
   d. ideal self.

2. Which of the following factors reinforces the development of a healthy self-concept?
   a. An individual accomplishes a goal.
   b. An individual experiences failure.
   c. Individuals avoid their cultural heritage.
   d. Individuals experience stress.

3. B.R., age 38, found a lump on her breast. Following a biopsy that confirmed the diagnosis of breast cancer, B.R. is scheduled for a mastectomy. She says that she will never look at such an ugly scar and that her husband will not love her anymore. Which of the following *nursing diagnoses* would be appropriate for the nurses to use?
   a. Disturbed **Body** Image
   b. Impaired **Coping**
   c. Risk for **Loneliness**
   d. Impaired Public **Image**

4. A 15-year-old male client tells the nurse, "I'm a scrawny, stupid loser." This statement best reflects the client's:
   a. real self
   b. other self
   c. public self
   d. ideal self

5. A 22-year-old female client is struggling with low self-esteem. Which of the following activities could the nurse teach the client to help increase her self-esteem?
   a. indulge her sweet tooth and eat a pint of ice cream
   b. make a list of all her flaws
   c. tell herself she's fine just as she is
   d. learn something new

# Spirituality

## Key Terms

Match the following terms with their correct definitions.

___ 1. Faith

___ 2. Hope

___ 3. Meditation

___ 4. Prayer

___ 5. Religion

___ 6. Spiritual distress

___ 7. Spirituality

___ 8. Transcendence

___ 9. Values

a. A state of being or existence above and beyond the limits of material experience.

b. Communication with spiritual and divine entities.

c. Activity that brings the mind and spirit in focus on the present.

d. Disruption in the life principle that pervades a person's entire well-being.

e. Looking forward with hope and confidence.

f. Principles, standards, or qualities considered worthwhile or desirable.

g. A system of organized beliefs, rituals, and wishes to be associated with.

h. Confident belief in the truth, values, or trustworthiness of a person, idea, or things.

i. Core of a person's being.

## Abbreviation Review

Write the meaning or definition of the following abbreviations, acronyms, and symbols.

1. ANA _____

2. NANDA _____

## Exercises and Activities

1. Explain the difference between prayer and meditation.

   _____

   _____

   _____

2. The client would like to learn about meditation. What are some of the basic steps to meditation?

_____

_____

_____

3. Describe the four ways in which parents transmit values to their children.

a. _____

b. _____

c. _____

d. _____

4. Discuss some of the ANA responsibilities for nurses who deal with spirituality issues.

_____

_____

_____

5. What are some of the defining characteristics of spiritual distress?

_____

_____

_____

6. Fill in the concept map for spiritual distress.

Connection to self

Connection with others

Nursing diagnosis: Spiritual Well-Being, Readiness for Enhanced

Connection with power greater than self

Connections with art, music, literature, or nature

## Self-Assessment Questions

Circle the letter that corresponds to the best answer.

1. The client is of the Jehovah's Witness faith. The nurse understands that which of the following options are contraindicated, as it would cause spiritual distress?
   a. Drinking coffee
   b. Receiving blood products
   c. Having surgery
   d. Eating pork products

2. An American Indian client uses cedar and sage as part of a ceremonial experience. How might the nurse make accommodations to the treatment plan in order to prevent spiritual distress with this client?
   a. Provide privacy for the ceremony.
   b. Ask to participate in the ceremony.
   c. Call the hospital chaplain for permission.
   d. Refuse to allow the ceremony to occur.

3. A new patient is being admitted to the nursing unit in the hospital. Which of the following questions helps the nurse determine if there are issues related to spirituality?
   a. When do you pray?
   b. Where do you pray?
   c. May I place your prayer beads in the bedside stand?
   d. What religious practices are important to you?

4. The client refuses to eat meat on certain days because of religious beliefs, yet the client needs protein for wound healing. How could the nurse resolve this dilemma?
   a. Insist the client eat the meat provided.
   b. Ask the dietician to help find other protein sources.
   c. Ask the family to bring food from home.
   d. Offer the client extra liquids on the special days.

5. The client who is dying of cancer states, " I wish God would just take me." This is an example of
   a. hope.
   b. values.
   c. spiritual distress.
   d. grief.

# Complementary/ Alternative Therapies

## Key Terms

Match the following terms with their correct definitions.

_____ 1. Acupressure

_____ 2. Acupuncture

_____ 3. Allopathic

_____ 4. Alternative therapies

_____ 5. Antioxidant

_____ 6. Aromatherapy

_____ 7. Biofeedback

_____ 8. Bodymind

_____ 9. Complementary therapies

_____ 10. Curing

_____ 11. Energy therapy

_____ 12. Free radical

_____ 13. Healing

a. Ridding of disease.

b. Altered state of consciousness or awareness resembling sleep and during which a person is more receptive to suggestion.

c. Folk healer-priest who uses natural and supernatural forces to help others.

d. Therapies used instead of conventional or mainstream medical practices.

e. Nonnutritive, physiologically active compounds present in plants in very small amounts; store nutrients and provide structure, aroma, flavor, and color.

f. Technique of releasing blocked energy within an individual when specific points (Tsubas) along the meridians are pressed or massaged by the practitioner's fingers, thumbs, and heel of the hands.

g. Measurement of physiological responses that yields information about the relationship between the mind and body and helps clients learn the way to manipulate these responses through mental activity.

h. Energy-based therapeutic modality that alters the energy fields through the use of touch, thereby affecting physical, mental, emotional, and spiritual health.

i. Quieting of the mind by focusing the attention.

j. Relaxation technique of using the imagination to visualize a pleasant, soothing image.

k. Therapies used in conjunction with conventional medical therapies.

l. Therapeutic use of concentrated essences or essential oils that have been extracted from plants and flowers.

m. Technique of application of heat and needles to various points on the body to alter the energy flow.

___14. Healing touch

___15. Hypnosis

___16. Imagery

___17. Meditation

___18. Neuropeptide

___19. Neurotransmitter

___20. Phytochemical

___21. Psychoneuroimmunoendo-
crinology

___22. Shaman

___23. Shamanism

___24. Therapeutic massage

___25. Therapeutic touch

___26. Touch

n. Inseparable connection and operation of thoughts, feelings, and physiological functions.

o. Amino acids produced in the brain and other sites in the body that act as chemical communicators.

p. Study of the complex relationship among the cognitive, affective, and physical aspects of humans.

q. Application of pressure and motion by the hands with the intent of improving the recipient's well-being.

r. Unstable molecules that alter genetic codes and trigger the development of cancer growth in cells.

s. A technique of assessing alterations in a person's energy fields and using the hands to direct energy to achieve a balanced state.

t. Chemical substances produced by the body that facilitate nerve-impulse transmission.

u. Means of perceiving or experiencing through tactile sensation.

v. Practice of entering altered states of consciousness with the intent of helping others.

w. Substance that prevents or inhibits oxidation, a chemical process wherein a substance is joined to oxygen.

x. Techniques of using the hands to direct or redirect the flow of the body's energy fields and thus enhance balance within those fields.

y. Process that activates the individual's recovery forces from within.

z. Traditional medical and surgical treatment.

## Abbreviation Review

Write the meaning or definition of the following abbreviations.

1. AAT _____

2. CA _____

3. FDA _____

4. NCAAM _____

5. NHI _____

6. PMR _____

7. PNIE _____

## Exercises and Activities

1. How would you describe a nurse's role in complementary/alternative therapy?

   _____

   _____

   _____

   a. How would you explain the concept of the bodymind to another student?

   _____

   _____

2. For each of the following cultures, write a short description of its health perception and specific examples of modern therapies.

| Culture | Health Perception | Modern Therapies |
|---|---|---|
| Greek culture | | |
| Far East | | |
| China | | |
| India | | |

3. Differentiate the following terms: therapeutic massage; therapeutic touch; healing touch.

   a. List a benefit of each complementary/alternative therapy.

   (1) _____

   (2) _____

   (3) _____

4. List two primary benefits of each of the following complementary/alternative therapies and the types of conditions they may help.

| Therapy | | Primary Benefits | Types of Conditions |
|---|---|---|---|
| Guided imagery | (1) | | |
| | (2) | | |
| Biofeedback | (1) | | |
| | (2) | | |
| Yoga | (1) | | |
| | (2) | | |
| Shiatsu/acupressure | (1) | | |
| | (2) | | |

a. Using Table 17-3, Medicinal Value of Selected Herbs, name two herbs a holistic practitioner might use for each of these conditions.

Healing a wound: _____

Mild depression: _____

Headache: _____

Common cold/sinus congestion: _____

b. Why should nurses encourage their clients to reveal the use of herbs to their primary care provider?

_____

_____

5. You have been working as an LP/VN at a long-term care facility since your graduation 6 months ago. The facility is pleasant, nicely decorated, and home to 64 residents. You particularly enjoy caring for C.S., whose daughter and granddaughter visit twice a week. On her next visit, the daughter mentions how much her father enjoyed his dog at home, a black Labrador retriever. She asks if this facility ever thought about having a pet therapy program. Apparently, many long-term care facilities are using pet therapy with very good results. You mention it to the supervising nurse, who asks you to evaluate the idea.

a. In what ways might a pet therapy program benefit the clients in this facility?

_____

_____

b. What issues would you need to consider?

_____

_____

c. What other types of complementary therapies might you consider for this facility?

_____

_____

d. If this were a long-term care facility for sick children, what complementary therapies might be appropriate?

_____

_____

## Self-Assessment Questions

Circle the letter that corresponds to the best answer.

1. The use of complementary/alternative therapies is increasing because most are
   a. noninvasive and inexpensive.
   b. covered by insurance.
   c. easy to learn at home.
   d. spiritual in nature.

2. Because it deals with physiological, psychological, sociological, intellectual, and spiritual aspects of the individual, nursing can be described as
   a. comprehensive.
   b. complemental.
   c. humanistic.
   d. holistic.

3. The nurse explains that the benefits of meditation for the client include
   a. decreased oxygen consumption and blood pressure.
   b. enhanced stamina, agility, and balance.
   c. restoration of sensation and function.
   d. increased heart rate and lactic acid.

4. Chiropractic therapy is an example of which category of complementary/alternative intervention?
   a. Energetic touch
   b. Manipulative body based
   c. Mind/body therapy
   d. None of the above

5. Reflexology is a complementary/alternative therapy based on the
   a. shamanistic tradition.
   b. human energy fields.
   c. ancient healing arts.
   d. Ayurvedic system.

6. The nurse understands that massage therapy
   a. is also called therapeutic touch.
   b. is useful with clients from all cultural backgrounds.
   c. may be contraindicated in hypertension and diabetes.
   d. is a treatment modality specified in the Nursing Practice Act.

7. Which statement is *not* an assumption of therapeutic touch?
   a. A human being is a closed energy system.
   b. Anatomically, a human being is bilaterally symmetrical.
   c. Illness is a balance in an individual's energy field.
   d. Human beings cannot transcend their conditions of living.

8. What complementary/alternative therapy employs proper breathing, posture, and movement?
   a. Yoga therapy
   b. Chiropractic therapy
   c. Energy therapy
   d. Touch therapy

9. Contraindications for massage therapy are
   a. necrosis and stiffness.
   b. immobility and phlebitis.
   c. varicose veins and dermatitis.
   d. inflammation and stress.

10. Reflexology is the art and science of
    a. correcting areas of vertebral subluxation.
    b. releasing blocked energy within Tsubas.
    c. enervating the nerves in the feet.
    d. using the hands to realign the energy flow.

# Basic Nutrition

## Key Terms

Match the following terms with their correct definitions.

___ 1. Absorption

___ 2. Anabolism

___ 3. Anthropometric measurements

___ 4. Atherosclerosis

___ 5. Basal metabolism

___ 6. Body mass index

___ 7. Calorie

___ 8. Catabolism

___ 9. Cholesterol

___10. Chyme

___11. Complete protein

___12. Deglutition

___13. Dehydration

___14. Diet therapy

a. Constructive process of metabolism whereby new molecules are synthesized and new tissues are formed, as in growth and repair.

b. Vitamin requiring the presence of fats for its absorption from the gastrointestinal (GI) tract into the lymphatic system and for cellular metabolism: vitamins A, D, E, and K.

c. Pancreatic hormone that aids in the diffusion of glucose into the liver and muscle cells and in the synthesis of glycogen.

d. Measurement used to ascertain whether a person's weight is appropriate for height; calculated by dividing the weight in kilograms by the height in meters squared.

e. Protein containing all nine essential amino acids.

f. Coordinated, rhythmic, serial contraction of the smooth muscles of the gastrointestinal tract.

g. Lipid compound consisting of three fatty acids and a glycerol molecule.

h. Process whereby the end products of digestion pass through the epithelial membranes in the small and large intestines and into the blood or lymph system.

i. Equivalent to 1,000 calories.

j. Vitamin that must be ingested daily in normal quantities because it is not stored in the body: vitamins C and B-complex.

k. Chewing food into fine particles and mixing the food with enzymes in saliva.

l. Conversion of amino acids into glucose.

m. Measurements of the size, weight, and proportions of the body.

n. Swallowing of food.

___15. Dietary prescription/order

o. All of the processes (ingestion, digestion, absorption, metabolism, and elimination) involved in consuming and utilizing food for energy, maintenance, and growth.

___16. Digestion

p. Fingerlike projections that line the small intestine.

___17. Empty calories

q. Sum total of all the biological and chemical processes in the body as they relate to the use of nutrients in every body cell.

___18. Enriched

r. Lack of fluid in the tissues.

___19. Enteral nutrition

s. Feeding method, meaning both the ingestion of food orally and the delivery of nutrients through a GI tube, but generally meaning the latter.

___20. Euglycemia

t. Descriptor for food in which nutrients not naturally occurring in the food are added to it.

___21. Excretion

u. Lipoid composed of glycerol, fatty acids, and phosphorus; the structural component of cells.

___22. Extracellular fluid

v. Condition wherein blood glucose levels become too high as a result of the absence of insulin.

___23. Fat-soluble vitamin

w. Organic compound that is insoluble in water but soluble in organic solvents such as ether and alcohol; also known as fats.

___24. Fortified

x. Energy needed to maintain essential physiological functions such as respiration, circulation, and muscle tone, when a person is at complete rest physically, digestively, and mentally.

___25. Gluconeogenesis

y. Weight that is 20% or more above the ideal body weight.

___26. Glycogenesis

z. Feeling of fulfillment.

___27. Glycogenolysis

aa. Elimination of drugs or waste products from the body.

___28. Hypergylcemia

bb. Condition wherein blood glucose levels are exceedingly low.

___29. Hypoglycemia

cc. Acidic, semifluid paste found in the GI tract.

___30. Incomplete protein

dd. Chemical process of combining with oxygen.

___31. Ingestion

ee. Treating a disease or disorder with a special diet.

___32. Insensible water loss

ff. Protein with one or more of the essential amino acids missing.

___33. Insulin

gg. Cardiovascular disease of fatty deposits on the inner lining, the tunica intima, of vessel walls.

___34. Intracellular fluid

hh. Quantity of heat required to raise the temperature of 1 gram of water 1°C.

___35. Ketosis

ii. Condition wherein acids called ketones accumulate in the blood urine, upsetting the acid–base balance.

___36. Kilocalorie

jj. Order written by the physician for food, including liquids.

___37. Kwashiorkor

___38. Lipid

___39. Marasmus

___40. Mastication

___41. Metabolic rate

___42. Metabolism

___43. Monounsaturated fatty acid

___44. Nutrition

___45. Obesity

___46. Oxidation

___47. Parenteral nutrition

___48. Peristalsis

___49. Phospholipid

___50. Polyunsaturated fatty acid

___51. Satiety

___52. Sensible water loss

___53. Triglyceride

___54. Villi

___55. Vitamin

___56. Water-soluble vitamin

kk. The taking of food into the digestive tract, generally through the mouth.

ll. Fluid outside the cells, including plasma fluid, lymph, cerebrospinal fluid, interstitial fluid, and GI fluids.

mm. Destructive process of metabolism whereby tissues or substances are broken into their component parts.

nn. Conversion of glucose into glycogen.

oo. Sterol produced by the body and used in the synthesis of steroid hormones.

pp. Mechanical and chemical processes that convert nutrients into a physically absorbable state.

qq. Conversion of glycogen into glucose.

rr. Fluid within the cells.

ss. Feeding method whereby nutrients bypass the small intestine and enter the blood directly.

tt. Normal blood glucose level.

uu. Descriptor for food in which nutrients that were removed during processing are added back in.

vv. Calories that provide few nutrients.

ww. Rate of energy utilization in the body.

xx. Fluids we are not conscious of losing, such as fluid lost through normal respiration.

yy. Fluids we are aware of losing, such as fluid lost through urine.

zz. A condition that results from sudden or recent lack of protein-containing foods that manifests in the client as edema, painful skin lesions, and changes in the pigmentation of skin and hair.

aaa. A condition that afflicts very young children who lack protein, energy foods, vitamins, and minerals, observable in a client who has an emaciated look, dull and dry hair, and thin and wrinkled skin.

bbb. Foods in this category are nuts, fowl, and olive oil.

ccc. Foods in this category are fish, sunflower seeds, and spy-beans.

ddd. Substances that regulate body processes and are necessary for metabolism of fats, carbohydrates, and proteins.

# Abbreviation Review

Write the meaning or definition of the following abbreviations and symbols.

1. AI _____
2. BMI _____
3. CHO _____
4. CHON _____
5. CI _____
6. CNS _____
7. dL _____
8. DNA _____
9. DRI _____
10. EAR _____
11. ECF _____
12. FDA _____
13. Fe _____
14. ft _____
15. g _____
16. GI _____
17. I&O _____
18. ICF _____
19. in _____
20. $K^+$ _____
21. kcal _____
22. kg _____
23. lb _____
24. Mg _____
25. mg _____
26. mL _____
27. Na _____
28. NG _____
29. NLEA _____
30. NPO _____
31. oz _____
32. P _____
33. RBC _____
34. RDA _____
35. RNA _____
36. S _____
37. TF _____

38. TPN _____

39. UL _____

40. USDA _____

41. WBC _____

42. Zn _____

## Exercises and Activities

1. Label the food groups on the food guide pyramid and include the recommended number of servings.

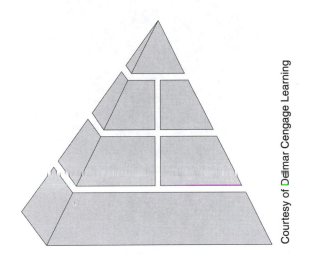

Courtesy of Delmar Cengage Learning

_____

_____

_____

_____

_____

_____

_____

a. Describe the role of the nurse in nutrition assessment.

_____

_____

_____

_____

b. Why is the role of education important in nutrition for clients?

_____

_____

_____

_____

2. Label the parts of the digestive system. Write a major function for each.

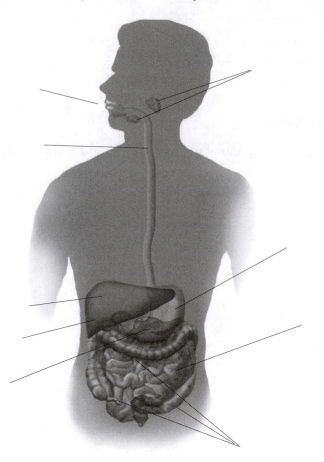

Courtesy of Delmar Cengage Learning

a. What is the function for each of these nutrients?

Water _____

Carbohydrates _____

Fats _____

Proteins _____

Vitamins _____

Minerals _____

3. Calculate the desired weight and caloric needs for each of the following clients.

a. The first client is a male who is 5 ft. 11 in. tall, with a large build.

Desired weight _____

Basal energy needs _____

This client's actual weight is 215 lb. What would be his actual basal energy needs?

Actual weight: 210 ÷ 2.2 = _____ kg

_____ kg × 1 × 24 = _____ basal kcal (basal energy needs)

He maintains a moderately active lifestyle. Determine his total energy requirements:

_____ (basal kcal) × _____ = _____ total kcal

Is this client considered obese? _____

b. Your second client is a female who is 5 ft. 2 in. tall, with a small build.

Desired weight _____

Basal energy needs _____

Her actual weight is 97 lb. Determine her actual basal energy needs.

Actual weight: 97 ÷ 2.2 = _____ kg

_____ kg × 1 × 24 = _____ basal kcal (basal energy needs)

She maintains a sedentary lifestyle. What are her total energy requirements?

_____ (basal kcal) × _____ = _____ total kcal

Is this client considered underweight? _____

4. List signs and symptoms of poor nutritional status in each of the following.

Skin: _____

_____

Hair: _____

_____

Nails: _____

_____

Eyes: _____

_____

Weight: _____

_____

Activity: _____

_____

a. What information would you include in a presentation to adolescents about healthy nutrition?

_____

_____

b. How do the physical changes of aging affect nutritional status in the older adult client?

_____

_____

c. List three interventions that can support a healthy nutritional intake for the older client.

(1) _____

(2) _____

(3) _____

d. How can an adequate caloric intake be maintained with the client who is unable to chew food or swallow well?

_____

_____

5. R.W., 29 years old, appears healthy and well nourished on her first prenatal visit. Her weight, at 134 lb., seems appropriate for her height of 5 ft. 4 in. Findings on her physical assessment indicate good nutritional status. She has been a vegetarian for 5 years and would like to know what adjustments she might need to her diet while she is pregnant.

a. Why is good nutrition important during pregnancy?

_____

_____

How many grams of protein are recommended for this client before pregnancy?

_____lb ÷ 2.2 lb/kg = _____kg

_____ kg × 0.8 g/kg = _____ gm protein/day

How does this requirement change for her pregnancy?

b. Describe one tool that could be used to assess her nutritional intake.

_____

_____

c. What items need to be included for a complete nutritional assessment for this client?

_____

_____

d. Describe any recommendations you would include for her vegetarian diet.

_____

_____

e. What information will you give R.W. about the benefits of lactation for her infant?

_____

_____

## Self-Assessment Questions

Circle the letter that corresponds to the best answer.

1. Signs of calcium deficiency include osteoporosis, tetany, poor tooth formation, and
   a. rickets.
   b. scurvy.
   c. anemia.
   d. pellagra.

2. Without sufficient carbohydrates, the body converts protein into glucose for energy. This process is called
   a. ketosis.
   b. catabolism.
   c. glycogenolysis.
   d. gluconeogenesis.

3. Which of the following statements is incorrect regarding nutrition needs for the older client?
   a. Calorie needs decrease about 2% to 3% every 10 years.
   b. Water requirements decrease along with fewer total calories.
   c. Canned foods should be avoided if there are cardiac problems.
   d. Protein requirements are stable, about 12% to 14% of total calories.

4. To ensure an adequate nutritional intake of zinc to promote wound healing, your client's diet should include
   a. meat, milk, and whole grains.
   b. bananas, oranges, and prunes.
   c. legumes, raisins, and apricots.
   d. legumes and green leafy vegetables.

5. The client with ulcerative colitis or Crohn's disease may be advised to avoid
   a. eggs, cheese, and milk.
   b. breads, cereal, and rice.
   c. raw fruits and whole grains.
   d. animal fats and milk products.

6. While caring for your client, you note decreased skin turgor, sunken eyes, and weight loss. Which of the following findings would the nurse anticipate?
   a. Increased venous filling times
   b. Decreased body temperature
   c. Increased protein intake
   d. Decreased urine output

7. The constructive process of metabolism is called
   a. catabolism.
   b. anabolism.
   c. oxidation.
   d. basal metabolism.

8. Inorganic nutrients include
   a. carbohydrates.
   b. fats.
   c. vitamins.
   d. minerals.

9. Which is *not* a source for sensible water loss?
   a. Urine
   b. Diarrhea
   c. Respiration
   d. Vomit

10. What type of carbohydrate requires no digestion and is quickly absorbed?
    a. Monosaccharides
    b. Disaccharides
    c. Polysaccharides
    d. Glycogen

# Rest and Sleep

## Key Terms

Match the following terms with their correct definitions.

___ 1. Biological clock

___ 2. Bruxism

___ 3. Cataplexy

___ 4. Chronobiology

___ 5. Circadian rhythm

___ 6. Hypersomnia

___ 7. Insomnia

___ 8. Narcolepsy

___ 9. Parasomnia

___10. REM disorder

___11. Rest

___12. Restless leg syndrome

___13. Sleep

___14. Sleep apnea

a. Alteration in sleep pattern characterized by excessive sleep, especially in the daytime.

b. Condition characterized by profoundly disturbed sleep due to behavioral or physiological events.

c. State of altered consciousness during which an individual experiences fluctuations in level of consciousness, minimal physical activity, and general slowing of the body's physiologic processes.

d. Grinding of teeth during sleep.

e. Syndrome wherein breathing periodically ceases during sleep for a period of 30 to 60 seconds; often associated with heavy snoring.

f. State of relaxation and calmness, both mental and physical.

g. Science of studying biorhythms.

h. Difficulty in falling asleep initially or in returning to sleep once awakened.

i. Sleep alteration manifested as sudden uncontrollable urges to fall asleep during the daytime.

j. Condition wherein the paralysis normally occurring during REM sleep is absent or incomplete and the sleeper acts out the dream that is occurring.

k. Condition characterized by uncomfortable sensations of tingling or crawling in the muscles, and twitching, burning, prickling, or deep aching in the foot, calf, or upper leg when at rest (lying or sitting).

l. Biorhythm that cycles on a daily basis.

m. Sudden loss of muscle control.

n. Internal mechanism capable of measuring time in a living organism.

___15. Sleep cycle

    o. Sleepwalking.

___16. Sleep deprivation

    p. Sequence of sleep that begins with the four stages of non–rapid eye movement sleep in order, with a return to stage 3 and then stage 2, followed by passage into the first rapid eye movement stage.

___17. Sleep hygiene

    q. Prolonged inadequate quality and quantity of sleep.

___18. Somnambulism

    r. Client's habits in preparing for sleep.

## Abbreviation Review

Write the meaning or definition of the following abbreviations and acronyms.

1. CPAP _____
2. EEG _____
3. NANDA _____
4. NREM _____
5. NSF _____
6. NSRED _____
7. PLMD _____
8. PMS _____
9. REM _____
10. RLS _____

## Exercises and Activities

1. Differentiate the terms *rest* and *sleep.* In what ways is each important to the health/wellness of an individual?

    _____
    _____
    _____

    a. What do you do at bedtime to help you sleep?

    _____
    _____

    b. In what ways, if any, has school affected your ability to rest or sleep?

    _____
    _____

    c. If you were hospitalized for a brief period, in what ways do you think it would affect your sleep patterns?

    _____
    _____

2. What impact might illness or the health care setting have on each of the following factors affecting sleep? List two interventions for each factor that could help promote rest/sleep for clients.

| Factor | Impact of Illness/Health Care | Interventions |
|---|---|---|
| Physical | | (1)<br>(2) |
| Psychological | | (1)<br>(2) |
| Environmental | | (1)<br>(2) |
| Lifestyle | | (1)<br>(2) |
| Diet | | (1)<br>(2) |

    a. What effect does medication have on rest and sleep?

3. Describe REM sleep. How does it differ from NREM sleep?

    a. What is the importance of adequate REM sleep for an individual?

    b. Describe the sleep pattern for a school-age child. What interventions might help the child to get adequate rest/sleep in a health care setting?

    c. Describe the sleep pattern for an older adult. What interventions might encourage rest and sleep in these clients?

4. L.P., a 68-year-old client, is scheduled for surgery in the morning. When you assessed him earlier, he seemed comfortable. You are making rounds again at 1 A.M. and you find him still awake. When you ask if he needs anything, L.P. assures you that he is fine, but he "just can't seem to get to sleep." You ask if he is having any pain, and he says he is fairly comfortable right now. After a little more discussion, you decide that he might be anxious about his surgery. You also note that his room seems a little warm, and his roommate, who is sleeping soundly, is also snoring loudly.

a. What nursing diagnosis might be appropriate for L.P.?

_____

_____

b. What factors could be interfering with his ability to sleep?

_____

_____

c. Describe interventions that you could use to encourage this client to sleep.

_____

_____

d. L.P. is being discharged home. When his wife arrives, she says, "At least I was able to get a little more sleep while he was in the hospital. He usually wakes me up several times a night at home." What questions might you want to ask his wife?

_____

_____

_____

## Self-Assessment Questions

Circle the letter that corresponds to the best answer.

1. Your client has a history of loud snoring, breathing pauses of 30 to 60 seconds, and daytime sleepiness. Based on this sleep assessment, your client may be experiencing
   a. narcolepsy.
   b. parasomnia.
   c. sleep apnea.
   d. hypersomnia.

2. A somnambulist is an individual who
   a. has difficulty falling asleep.
   b. has daytime sleepiness.
   c. treats sleep disorders.
   d. sleepwalks.

3. All but which of the following are treatments used for sleep apnea?
   a. Dental appliances
   b. Medication
   c. Surgery
   d. CPAP

4. The nurse is conducting a sleep assessment on an elderly client. The nurse understands that the client is at increased risk for
   a. restless leg syndrome.
   b. somnambulism.
   c. hypersomnia.
   d. sleep terrors.

5. The client with sleep apnea is at a greater risk for hypertension and
   a. narcolepsy.
   b. headache.
   c. bruxism.
   d. stroke.

6. A nurse who works on the night shift is at greater risk of sleep deprivation due to an alteration in
   a. environment.
   b. lifestyle.
   c. aging.
   d. diet.

7. Nearly half of normal adult NREM sleep is spent in
   a. stage 1.
   b. stage 2.
   c. stage 3.
   d. stage 4.

8. What food items frequently disrupt sleep?
   a. Alcohol and tea
   b. Spicy foods and chips
   c. Cola and snacks
   d. Chocolate and coffee

9. A medication that may cause insomnia is
   a. hydroxyzine.
   b. diphenhydramine.
   c. captopril.
   d. amitriptyline.

10. The hallmark symptom of narcolepsy is
    a. cataplexy.
    b. snoring.
    c. leg movements.
    d. bruxism.

# Safety/Hygiene

## Key Terms

Match the following terms with their correct definitions.

____ 1. Body image

____ 2. Chemical restraint

____ 3. Dental caries

____ 4. Gingivitis

____ 5. Halitosis

____ 6. Hygiene

____ 7. Perineal care

____ 8. Physical restraint

____ 9. Poison

____10. Pyorrhea

____11. Restraint

____12. Self-care deficit

____13. Sensory overload

____14. Stomatitis

a. Periodontal disease.

b. Science of health.

c. Cavities.

d. Individual's perception of physical self, including appearance, function, and ability.

e. Inflammation of the gums.

f. Increased perception of the intensity of auditory and visual stimuli.

g. Any substance that when taken into the body interferes with normal physiologic functioning; may be inhaled, injected, ingested, or absorbed by the body.

h. Bad breath.

i. State wherein an individual is not able to perform one or more activities of daily living.

j. Medication used to control client behavior.

k. Cleansing of the external genitalia and perineum and the surrounding area.

l. Protective device used to limit the physical activity of a client or to immobilize a client or extremity.

m. Inflammation of the oral mucosa.

n. Equipment that reduces the client's movement.

## Abbreviation Review

Write the meaning or definition of the following abbreviations and acronyms.

1. ADL _____

2. CDC _____

3. CHD _____

4. CMS _____

5. CPR _____

6. FDA _____

7. GCS _____

8. HDL _____

9. ID _____

10. JCAHO _____

11. MSDS _____

12. NANDA _____

13. OBRA _____

14. OSHA _____

15. PCA _____

## Exercises and Activities

1. Why is safety an important issue for clients?

   _____

   _____

   _____

   a. Why is safety important for health care workers?

   _____

   _____

   b. In what ways does OSHA assist health care workers?

   _____

   _____

   c. Explain right-to-know laws.

   _____

   _____

   d. What is contained on a material safety data sheet?

   _____

   _____

2. You have been asked to help with orientation for new nursing students at your facility. What would you include in a safety presentation to them? Include safety measures for clients and for the nursing students.

   _____

   _____

   _____

   _____

   _____

   _____

a.  What safety instructions would you give to a client who has recently been admitted to your facility?

_____

_____

3.  Why is fire such a serious risk in a health care facility?

_____

_____

_____

a.  List five interventions that can prevent or reduce the risk of fire in the health care setting.

(1) _____

(2) _____

(3) _____

(4) _____

(5) _____

b.  What would you do if a fire were discovered?

_____

_____

4.  Describe risk factors and list three interventions for each developmental age to facilitate safety.

| Developmental Age | Risk Factors | Interventions |
| --- | --- | --- |
| Infant/toddler | | (1)<br>(2)<br>(3) |
| School-age child | | (1)<br>(2)<br>(3) |
| Adolescent | | (1)<br>(2)<br>(3) |
| Adult | | (1)<br>(2)<br>(3) |

a.  How does the aging process affect a client's safety?

_____

_____

b.  In what ways does proper hygiene promote health or healing for the client?

_____

_____

5.  S.J. is an 83-year-old client with a history of congestive heart failure and pneumonia that has resolved. She is also healing from a right hip fracture that resulted from a fall at home. Medications include a diuretic and occasional mild analgesic for pain. S.J. responds slowly when you try to get her attention and is often confused about where she is. Her appetite is usually poor, but she will take about half her food with some encouragement. Caregivers refer to her as "frail" and have noted reddened areas over her back and left ankle. Although she is in a wheelchair for part of the day, she has lost strength and mobility in her legs and spends most of her time in bed. She is usually incontinent.

a.  Evaluate S.J.'s risk status for skin integrity using Table 20-1 in your text.

_____

_____

b.  What fall risk factors are present for this client?

_____

_____

c.  List several interventions that could protect S.J. from injury.

(1) _____

(2) _____

(3) _____

(4) _____

(5) _____

(6) _____

(7) _____

(8) _____

d.  Restraints have been ordered for S.J. to be used during the night. What special precautions must be taken?

_____

_____

e.  You are prepared to medicate S.J. and discover that she has no identification band. How would you proceed?

_____

_____

f.  If S.J. were to be transferred to home care with portable oxygen, what safety advice would you give to her family?

_____

_____

## Self-Assessment Questions

Circle the letter that corresponds to the best answer.

1. The nurse discovers a fire in a client's room. The first priority for the nurse is
   a. ensuring the client's safety.
   b. calling the fire department.
   c. trying to extinguish the fire.
   d. closing doors to other rooms.

2. A client with wrist restraints in place must be assessed at least every 2 hours for
   a. vital signs.
   b. range of motion.
   c. proper body mechanics.
   d. circulation and sensation.

3. Which of the following statements is correct regarding personal hygiene of the client?
   a. Gloves are not needed for bathing a client.
   b. It is best when performed by nursing staff.
   c. Clients should be encouraged to perform their own perineal care.
   d. Reddened areas on the skin should be massaged during the bath.

4. Assessment of the client's hair during shampoo and combing can provide information about the client's
   a. skin integrity.
   b. medication use.
   c. fall risk potential.
   d. general health status.

5. Periodontal disease can be prevented through
   a. regular dental care.
   b. good oral hygiene.
   c. using fluoride drops.
   d. massaging the gums.

6. The organization that outlines and enforces regulations that all health facilities must follow with regard to employees and exposure to and handling of potentially infectious materials is
   a. MSDS.
   b. CDC.
   c. OSHA.
   d. FDA.

7. What is it called when a client is not able to perform one or more activities of living?
   a. Risk for injury
   b. Personal preference
   c. Precautionary feedback
   d. Self-care deficit

8. All are safe alternatives to side-rail use except
   a. a low-height bed.
   b. a bed mats.
   c. a bed alarm.
   d. a motion sensor.

9. An alternative to restraint use is
   a. placing the call light in reach.
   b. providing bathroom breaks every 4 hours.
   c. removing extra pillows and blankets.
   d. maintaining the hospital schedule.

10. What type of fire extinguisher would you use for an electrical fire?
    a. Class A
    b. Class B
    c. Class C
    d. Class D

# Infection Control/ Asepsis

## Key Terms

Match the following terms with their correct definitions.

___ 1. Acquired immunity

___ 2. Agent

X 3. Airborne transmission

___ 4. Antibody

H 5. Asepsis

rf 6. Aseptic technique

___ 7. Bactericide

___ 8. Biological agent

___ 9. Carrier

___10. Chain of infection

___11. Chemical agent

q 12. Clean object

___13. Cleansing

a. Transfer of an agent to a susceptible host by animate means such as mosquitoes, fleas, ticks, lice, and other animals.

b. Practices that reduce the number, growth, and spread of microorganisms.

c. Microorganisms that occur or have adapted to live in a specific environment, such as intestinal, skin, vaginal, or oral flora.

d. Formation of antibodies (memory B cells) to protect against future invasions of an already experienced antigen.

e. Physical transfer of an agent from an infected person to a host through direct contact with that person, indirect contact with an infected person through a fomite, or close contact with contaminated secretions.

f. Process of invasion by and multiplication of pathogenic microorganisms that occurs in body tissue and results in cellular injury.

g. Practices that eliminate all microorganisms and spores from an object or area.

h. Transfer of an agent to a susceptible host by contaminated inanimate objects such as food, milk, drugs, and blood.

i. Route by which an infectious agent enters the host.

j. Object contaminated with an infectious agent.

k. Phenomenon of the development of an infectious process.

l. Infection that was acquired in a hospital or other health care facility and was not present or incubating at the time of the client's admission.

m. Microorganisms that attach to the skin for a brief period of time but do not continuously live on the skin.

____14. Colonization

____15. Communicable agent

____16. Communicable disease

____17. Compromised host

____18. Contact transmission

____19. Dirty object

____20. Disinfectant

____21. Disinfection

____22. Edema

____23. Erythema

____24. Flora

____25. Fomite

____26. Germicide

____27. Hand hygiene

____28. Hospital-acquired infection

____29. Host

____30. Humoral immunity

____31. Immunization

____32. Incubation period

____33. Infection

____34. Infectious agent

____35. Inflammation

____36. Localized infection

____37. Medical asepsis

____38. Mode of transmission

n. Frequency with which a pathogen causes disease.

o. Microorganisms that are always present, usually without altering the client's health.

p. Rubbing together of all surfaces and crevices of the hands using a soap or chemical and water, followed by rinsing in a flowing stream of water.

q. Object on which there are microorganisms that are usually not pathogenic.

r. Disease caused by a communicable agent.

s. Microorganism that causes disease.

t. Person who lacks resistance to an agent and is thus vulnerable to disease.

u. Infectious agent transmitted to a client by direct or indirect contact, via vehicle, vector, or airborne route.

v. Chemical that can be applied to both animate and inanimate objects for the purpose of eliminating pathogens.

w. Multiplication of microorganisms that occurs on or within a host but does not result in cellular injury.

x. Transfer of an agent to a susceptible host through droplet nuclei or dust particles suspended in the air.

y. Person whose normal defense mechanisms are impaired and who is therefore susceptible to infection.

z. Bacteria-killing chemicals found in tears.

aa. Simple or complex organism that can be affected by an agent.

bb. Inoculation with a vaccine to produce immunity against specific diseases.

cc. Infection limited to a defined area or single organ.

dd. Place where the agent can survive.

ee. Total elimination of all microorganisms, including spores.

ff. Object on which there is a high number of microorganisms, some of which are potentially pathogenic.

gg. Process of creating immunity or resistance to infection in an individual.

hh. Removal of soil or organic material from instruments and equipment used in providing client care.

ii. Protein substance that counteracts and neutralizes the effects of antigens and destroys bacteria and other cells.

jj. Detectable accumulation of increased interstitial fluid.

kk. Stimulation of B cells and antibody production.

ll. Process that bridges the gap between the portal of exit of the infectious agent from the reservoir or source and the portal of entry of the susceptible "new" host.

___39. Nosocomial infection

___40. Pathogen

___41. Pathogenicity

___42. Physical agent

___43. Portal of entry

___44. Portal of exit

___45. Reservoir

___46. Resident flora

___47. Sterilization

___48. Surgical asepsis

___49. Susceptible host

___50. Systemic infection

___51. Transient flora

___52. Vaccination

___53. Vector-borne transmission

___54. Vehicle transmission

___55. Virulence

mm. Microorganism that causes infection.

nn. Route by which an infectious agent leaves the reservoir.

oo. Entity capable of causing disease.

pp. Substance that interacts with a host, causing disease.

qq. Person who harbors an infectious agent but has no symptoms of disease.

rr. Infection control practice used to prevent the transmission of pathogens.

ss. Chemical solution used to clean inanimate objects.

tt. Absence of microorganisms.

uu. Infection that affects the entire body with involvement of multiple organs.

vv. Nonspecific cellular response to tissue injury.

ww. Ability of a microorganism to produce disease.

xx. Increased blood flow to an inflamed area.

yy. Factor in the environment capable of causing disease in a host.

zz. Elimination of pathogens, with the exception of spores, from inanimate objects.

aaa. Living organism that invades a host, causing disease.

bbb. Nosocomal infection.

ccc. Time interval between entry of an infectious agent in the host and the onset of symptoms.

## Abbreviation Review

Write the meaning or definition of the following abbreviations, acronyms, and symbols.

1. AIDS _____

2. APIC _____

3. CDC _____

4. DNA _____

5. EPA _____

6. ESR _____

7. HBV _____

8. HCV _____

9. HIV _____

10. NANDA _____

11. OR _____

12. OSHA _____

13. pH _____

14. RNA _____

15. TB _____

16. WBC _____

## Exercises and Activities

1. Differentiate the terms *infection* and *inflammation*.

   _____

   _____

   _____

   a. Briefly describe the five stages of the inflammatory process.

      (1) _____

      (2) _____

      (3) _____

      (4) _____

      (5) _____

   b. Describe each of the four stages of the infection process.

      (1) _____

      (2) _____

      (3) _____

      (4) _____

   c. How would you explain nosocomial infection to another student?

      _____

      _____

2. Match the essential element on the left with its appropriate location in the diagram.

Source

Biological agent

Susceptible host

Mode of transmission

Portal of entry to host

Portal of exit from source

Courtesy of Delmar Cengage Learning

a. Give one specific method to break the chain of infection among the preceding links for the common cold virus.

_____

_____

b. What makes hand hygiene the first line of defense for infection control?

_____

_____

c. Describe several characteristics that make an individual a more susceptible host for infections.

_____

_____

_____

_____

3. In what way is education important for prevention of disease

a. for health care workers?

_____

_____

b. for clients and family members?

_____

_____

c. You are preparing to talk to the parents of a 5-year-old child who will be attending school. What suggestions can you include about preventing infection and disease (immunizations, staying healthy, avoiding spread of illness, and so on)?

_____

_____

_____

_____

4. A.W. is a 77-year-old client admitted to a long-term care facility following several small strokes that have affected her ability to speak and swallow. Her nurse notes that A.W.'s nutritional status is poor, and she appears to have difficulty coughing up secretions effectively. Her activity level has greatly diminished, and she spends most of her time in bed. The nurse is concerned because several visitors and staff members have recently become ill with a flu virus.

a. What factors make this client a more susceptible host for disease?

_____

_____

b. List two nursing diagnoses for A.W..

(1) _____

(2) _____

c. How can this client strengthen her immune system?

_____

_____

d. Identify possible fomites in this health care environment.

_____

_____

## Self-Assessment Questions

Circle the letter that corresponds to the best answer for each question.

1. Chemical agents that can cause disease include pesticides, food additives, and
   a. spores.
   b. fomites.
   c. radiation.
   d. medications.

2. The most effective way to reduce the incidence of nosocomial infection is for health care workers to
   a. use germicide solutions on all surfaces.
   b. wash hands frequently and thoroughly.
   c. understand the chain of infection transmission.
   d. use aseptic technique with all medical procedures.

3. The nurse notes that the client has a low-grade fever and fatigue following exposure to the measles virus. The nurse understands that the client
   a. will be contagious within 3 days.
   b. is in the incubation period of the disease.
   c. is in the prodromal phase and is contagious.
   d. is in the illness stage, with signs and symptoms of measles.

4. A nurse is preparing to perform a urinary catheterization on a client. For this procedure, the nurse will
   a. maintain a sterile field and surgical asepsis.
   b. use gowning and a closed gloving technique.
   c. dispose of wastes in a sharps-disposal container.
   d. perform the catheterization using medical aseptic technique.

5. A mother is requesting antibiotics to treat a sore throat and cough in her 5-year-old child. The use of antibiotics may be discouraged for which of the following reasons?
   a. The child is too young to benefit from antibiotics.
   b. Antibiotics may impair the child's natural immunity.
   c. The medication may not be covered by health insurance.
   d. Antibiotics destroy normal flora and may not be effective.

6. Microorganisms that are always present are called
   a. resident flora.
   b. pathogens.
   c. bacteria.
   d. viruses.

7. Organisms that can live only inside the cell are called
   a. resident flora.
   b. pathogens.
   c. bacteria.
   d. viruses.

8. All of the following are types of agents capable of causing disease except
   a. bacteria and heat.
   b. pesticides and light.
   c. viruses and fomites.
   d. fungi and medication.

9. Which is *not* an example of a contact mode of transmission?
   a. Secretion from a client
   b. Coughing
   c. Bathing
   d. Specimen containers

10. An example of a specific immune defense is
    a. an antibody
    b. skin
    c. mucous membrane
    d. inflammation

# Standard Precautions and Isolation

---

## Key Terms

Match the following terms with their correct definitions.

_c_ 1. Airborne Precautions

_i_ 2. Aseptic Technique

___ 3. Barrier Precautions

_d_ 4. Contact Precautions

_f_ 5. Droplet Precautions

___ 6. Endemic

___ 7. Epidemic

___ 8. Hospital-acquired infection

___ 9. Isolation

_b_ 10. Reverse isolation

a. Separate from other persons, especially those with infectious diseases.

b. Barrier protection designed to prevent infection in clients who are severely compromised and highly susceptible to infection; also known as protective isolation.

c. Measures taken in addition to Standard Precautions and for clients known to have or suspected of having illnesses spread by airborne droplet nuclei.

d. Measures taken in addition to Standard Precautions and for clients known to have or suspected of having illnesses easily spread by direct client contact or contact with fomites.

e. Practices designed for clients documented as or suspected of being infected with highly transmissible or epidemiologically important pathogens for which additional precautions beyond the Standard Precautions are required to interrupt transmission in hospitals.

f. Measures taken in addition to Standard Precautions and for clients known to have or suspected of having serious illnesses spread by large-particle droplets.

g. Infection that is acquired in the hospital and was not present or incubating at the time of the client's admission.

h. Occurring continuously in a particular population and having low mortality.

i. Infection control practice used to prevent the transmission of pathogens.

j. Preventive practices to be used in the care of all clients in hospitals regardless of diagnosis or presumed infection status.

___11.  Standard Precautions

k.  Use of personal protective equipment, such as masks, gowns, and gloves, to create a barrier between the person and the microorganisms and thus prevent transmission of the microorganism.

___12.  Transmission-Based Precautions

l.  Infecting many people at the same time and in the same geographic area.

## Abbreviation Review

Write the meaning or definition of the following abbreviations and acronyms.

1. AIDS _____

2. BSI _____

3. CDC _____

4. DHHS _____

5. HBV _____

6. HICPAC _____

7. HIV _____

8. MDR _____

9. OSHA _____

10. TB _____

## Exercises and Activities

1. In what ways have infection control practices changed since 1985?

   _____

   _____

   _____

   a.  What is the purpose of the Hospital Infection Control Practices Advisory Committee?

   _____

   _____

2. What is the role of the nurse in preventing the spread of nosocomial infections?

   _____

   _____

   _____

   a.  List five actions or techniques to help reduce your occupational exposure to infection and disease.

   (1) _____

   (2) _____

   (3) _____

   (4) _____

   (5) _____

b. How does reverse isolation protect clients who are highly susceptible to infection?

_____

_____

3. Describe Standard Precautions.

_____

_____

_____

a. How do Standard Precautions differ from Universal Precautions?

_____

_____

b. Why were Transmission-Based Precautions added to Standard Precautions for infection control procedures?

_____

_____

c. Describe each of the following types of Transmission-Based Precautions:

Airborne Precautions: _____

_____

Contact Precautions: _____

_____

Droplet Precautions: _____

_____

d. Which type of precautions would be appropriate for each of the following diseases?
   (1) Airborne
   (2) Contact
   (3) Droplet
   _____ Pneumonia
   _____ Chickenpox
   _____ Scarlet fever
   _____ Scabies
   _____ Measles
   _____ Rubella
   _____ Impetigo
   _____ Meningitis

4. E.Y. is a 74-year-old client who was hospitalized for several days for treatment of dehydration and a gastrointestinal disorder. He is now improving his hydration and nutrition status but has been developing a pressure ulcer on his right buttock. The nurse caring for E.Y. today notes that the wound is open and draining. The drainage from the wound appears purulent and has a foul odor.

a. What types of precautions should be followed in providing this client's care?

_____

_____

b. Describe barrier precautions that will be used by E.Y.'s nurse.

_____

_____

c. If gloves are used while providing care for E.Y., why is hand hygiene still essential?

_____

_____

d. Do family members need to follow any special precautions while visiting E.Y.?

_____

_____

e. How would you address family members' concerns about why this client is now being "isolated."

_____

_____

## Self-Assessment Questions

Circle the letter that corresponds to the best answer.

1. The primary impact of the CDC guidelines in 1970 and 1975 was to
   a. introduce Body Substance Isolation.
   b. determine seven categories of isolation.
   c. establish Blood and Body Fluid Precautions.
   d. allow users to decide which guideline was appropriate for a given situation.

2. The most important and basic aspect of Standard Precautions is to
   a. know the medical diagnosis.
   b. limit contact with the client.
   c. wash hands frequently.
   d. use gown and gloves.

3. A nurse is caring for a client who is suspected of having pulmonary tuberculosis. The nurse will use personal protective equipment that includes
   a. goggles.
   b. sterile gloves.
   c. a surgical mask.
   d. an N95 respirator.

4. The nurse caring for a client diagnosed with varicella zoster (shingles) will use
   a. Contact Precautions.
   b. Universal Precautions.
   c. barrier nursing procedures.
   d. a negative air pressure room.

5. The nurse is most likely to use reverse isolation with a client who
   a.  has a latex allergy.
   b.  is immunocompromised because of chemotherapy.
   c.  requires multiple medical procedures.
   d.  may have a serious undiagnosed disease.

6. A client is noted to have purulent drainage from a wound. The nurse caring for this client will first
   a.  tell the client about precautions to take at home.
   b.  encourage all personnel to use good hand hygiene.
   c.  institute appropriate precautions and obtain a culture.
   d.  speak with the physician the next day about precautions.

7. According to OSHA regulations, all health care facilities must provide
   a.  hepatitis B vaccine at a minimal charge.
   b.  protective equipment.
   c.  training about occupational exposure every 2 years.
   d.  containers for sharps disposal every 6 feet.

8. Used needles can only be:
   a.  capped using the one-handed "scoop" technique.
   b.  recapped using both hands.
   c.  broken for disposal.
   d.  thrown away.

9. What is the appropriate type of precaution for a client with diphtheria? _chickenpox?_
   a.  Airborne
   b.  Contact
   c.  Droplet
   d.  Precautions are not needed for this client.

10. Which is *not* a psychological intervention for the client in isolation?
    a.  Encouraging verbalization of feelings
    b.  Encouraging visitors with appropriate barrier precautions
    c.  Supporting existing coping mechanisms
    d.  Discussing with team members the isolation process

# Bioterrorism

## Key Terms

Match the following terms with their correct definitions.

___ 1. Anthrax

___ 2. Bioterrorism

___ 3. Centers for Disease Control and Prevention

___ 4. Chemical, Biological, Radiological, Nuclear, and Explosive Enhanced Response Force Packages

___ 5. Chemical warfare agent

___ 6. Expeditionary medical support

___ 7. First responders

___ 8. Nerve agents

___ 9. Plague

___10. Radiation sickness

___11. Ricin

___12. Sarin

___13. Smallpox

___14. Terrorism

___15. Zoonotic disease

a. A highly contagious and frequently fatal viral disease.

b. Using any product, weapon, or threat of using a harmful act or substance to kill or injure others.

c. Disease caused by *Bacillus anthracis* bacteria.

d. A total package that includes everything necessary to screen and treat clients.

e. Poison made from castor beans.

f. Result of exposure to ionizing radiation.

g. EMEDS package plus a surgical suite.

h. Fast-acting clear, colorless, tasteless gas.

i. First people who respond to emergency situations.

j. Powerful acetycholinesterase inhibitors.

k. Gases, liquids, or solids that cause injury and death to people, plants, or animals.

l. Federal agency whose goal is to promote health and quality of life.

m. Purposeful use of biological agents for the purpose of harming, killing, and/or instilling fear.

n. Infection caused by the *Yersina pestis* bacteria.

o. Disease of animals that is directly transmissible to humans from the primary animal host.

## Abbreviation Review

Write the meaning or definition of the following abbreviations and acronyms.

1. CDC  _____

2. CERFPS  _____

3. EMEDS _____

4. EOP _____

5. FEMA _____

6. KI _____

7. SNS _____

8. VMI _____

9. VX _____

## Exercises and Activities

1. Using Table 23–1 in the text as a reference, describe the three categories of biological agents.

   Category A _____

   Category B _____

   Category C _____

2. Why are biological agents advantageous to use as a weapon?

   _____

   _____

   _____

3. E.C. is a dairy farmer in an area of the Upper Midwest that has naturally occurring anthrax bacteria. What are the three forms of human anthrax?

   _____

   _____

   _____

   a. Explain the most likely cause of E.C.'s anthrax disease.

   _____

   _____

   b. Why is exposure to anthrax spores a particular problem?

   _____

   _____

   c. Why would E.C.'s case not be considered terrorism?

   _____

   _____

   d. If E.C. develops cutaneous anthrax, describe what the lesions look like.

   _____

   _____

   e. What antibiotics would E.C. be most likely to receive if he had no known drug allergies?

   _____

   _____

4. Explain how the smallpox virus causes infection.

_____

_____

_____

  a. Describe the symptoms of smallpox.

  _____

  _____

  b. If smallpox can be prevented by vaccination, explain why mass vaccinations are no longer
     recommended.

  _____

  _____

  c. What precautions would a nurse need to make if a client were diagnosed with smallpox?

  _____

  _____

5. Plague is considered to be a zoonotic disease. What does this mean?

_____

_____

_____

  a. How is the transmission of bubonic and pneumonic plague different?

  _____

  _____

  b. How would a terrorist use the plague bacteria as a weapon?

  _____

  _____

  c. How soon should antibiotics be administered to a plague victim?

  _____

  _____

6. Identify chemicals that could be used for terrorism.

_____

_____

_____

  a. What was the intended use of chemical agents introduced in World War I?

  _____

  _____

7. Explain the role of FEMA in a bioterrorism event.

_____

_____

_____

8. How does the Strategic National Stockpile work?

_____

_____

_____

## Self-Assessment Questions

Circle the letter that corresponds to the best answer.

1. If a terrorist group uses sarin as a weapon, which actions would a first responder take first?
   a. Move the victims into fresh air.
   b. Remove the contaminated clothing.
   c. Flush the exposed area with copious amounts of water.
   d. Induce vomiting.

2. Following the atomic bomb in Hiroshima, Japan, in World War II, those that were exposed to high doses of radiation developed
   a. skin cancers.
   b. leukemia.
   c. pneumonia.
   d. heart attacks.

3. Potassium iodide (KI) is given in the event of a nuclear explosion. Which of the following is true of KI usage?
   a. It prevents lung cancer.
   b. It prevents radioactive iodine from entering the thyroid gland.
   c. KI protects all the organs of the endocrine system.
   d. It must be taken for two weeks following exposure.

4. JCAHO requires hospitals to have Emergency Operations Plan. What is contained in an Emergency Operations Plan?
   a. Information on how to activate the plan
   b. Who to notify at federal levels
   c. Who to notify at state levels
   d. Which security personnel to call

5. A nurse is caring for a patient who developed anthrax in the respiratory form. What precautions should the nurse take for herself?
   a. Standard precautions when working with bodily fluids.
   b. No precautions necessary, as it is not contagious in the respiratory form
   c. Strict isolation
   d. Respiratory precautions

# Fluid, Electrolyte, and Acid–Base Balance

## Key Terms

Match the following terms with their correct definitions.

___ 1. Acid

___ 2. Acidosis

___ 3. Alkalosis

___ 4. Anion

___ 5. Arterial blood gases

___ 6. Atom

___ 7. Base

___ 8. Buffer

___ 9. Cation

___ 10. Compound

___ 11. Crenation

___ 12. Decomposition

___ 13. Dehydration

___ 14. Dialysis

___ 15. Diffusion

___ 16. Edema

a. Decreased oxygen level in the blood.

b. Pressure that a fluid exerts against a membrane; also called filtration force.

c. Solution that has the same molecular concentration as does the cell; also called an isosmolar solution.

d. Substances combined in no specific way.

e. Measurement of levels of oxygen, carbon dioxide, pH, partial pressure of oxygen, partial pressure of carbon dioxide, saturation of oxygen, and bicarbonate in arterial blood.

f. Substance that attempts to maintain pH range, or hydrogen ion concentration, in the presence of added acids or bases.

g. Condition wherein cells decrease in size, shrivel and wrinkle, and are no longer functional when in a hypertonic solution.

h. Condition wherein more water is lost from the body than is replaced.

i. Seepage of fluid into the interstitial tissue as a result of accidental dislodgement of the IV needle from the vein.

j. Pressure exerted against the cell membrane by the water inside a cell.

k. Membrane that allows passage of only certain substances.

l. Normal resiliency of the skin.

m. Equilibrium (balance); consistency of body fluids.

n. Rupture of red blood cells due to osmosis.

o. Administration of fluids, electrolytes, nutrients, or medications by the venous route.

p. Fluid in tissue spaces around each cell.

\_\_\_\_17. Electrolyte

q. Measurement of the total concentration of dissolved particles (solutes) per kilogram of water.

\_\_\_\_18. Element

r. Diffusion used to separate molecules out of a solution by passing them through a semipermeable membrane.

\_\_\_\_19. Extracellular fluid

s. Substance that when dissociated produces ions that will combine with hydrogen ions.

\_\_\_\_20. Filtration

t. Condition characterized by an excessive number of hydrogen ions in a solution.

\_\_\_\_21. Hemolysis

u. In a solution, liquid, or gas, movement of molecules from an area of high molecular concentration to one of low molecular concentration.

\_\_\_\_22. Homeostasis

v. Element or compound that, when dissolved in water or another solvent, dissociates (separates) into ions (electrically charged particles).

\_\_\_\_23. Hydrostatic pressure

w. Fluid within the cells.

\_\_\_\_24. Hypertonic solution

x. Atoms of the same element that have different atomic weights (i.e., different numbers of neutrons in the nucleus).

\_\_\_\_25. Hypotonic solution

y. Product formed when an acid and a base react with each other.

\_\_\_\_26. Hypoxemia

z. Concentration of solutes per liter of cellular fluid.

\_\_\_\_27. Infiltration

aa. Anything that occupies space and possesses mass.

\_\_\_\_28. Interstitial fluid

bb. Ion bearing a positive charge.

\_\_\_\_29. Intracellular fluid

cc. Condition characterized by an excessive loss of hydrogen ions from a solution.

\_\_\_\_30. Intravascular fluid

dd. Smallest unit of an element that still retains the properties of that element that cannot be altered by any chemical change.

\_\_\_\_31. Intravenous therapy

ee. Detectable accumulation of increased interstitial fluid.

\_\_\_\_32. Ion

ff. Solution that has a lower molecular concentration than the cell; also called hypo-osmolar solution.

\_\_\_\_33. Isotonic solution

gg. Process of fluids and the substances dissolved in them being forced through the cell membrane by hydrostatic pressure.

\_\_\_\_34. Isotopes

hh. Diffusion from a region of higher concentration to a region of lower concentration.

\_\_\_\_35. Matter

ii. Joined with oxygen.

\_\_\_\_36. Mixture

jj. Chemical reaction when two or more atoms, called reactants, bond and form a more complex molecular product.

\_\_\_\_37. Molecule

kk. Fluid outside of the cells; includes interstitial, intravascular, synovial, cerebrospinal, and serous fluids; aqueous and vitreous humor; and endolymph and perilymph.

___38. Osmolality

___39. Osmolarity

___40. Osmosis

___41. Osmotic pressure

___42. Oxidized

___43. Permeability

___44. Potential hydrogen (pH)

___45. Salt

___46. Semipermeable membrane

___47. Synthesis

___48. Turgor

ll. Fluid consisting of the plasma in the blood vessels and the lymph in the lymphatic system.

mm. Atoms of the same element that unite with each other.

nn. Ability of a membrane to permit substances to pass through it.

oo. Any substance that in a solution yields hydrogen ions bearing a positive charge.

pp. Ion bearing a negative charge.

qq. Combination of atoms of two or more elements.

rr. Chemical reaction wherein the bonding between atoms in a molecule is broken and simpler products are formed.

ss. Solution that has a higher molecular concentration than the cell; also called a hyperosmolar solution.

tt. Basic substance of matter.

uu. Atom bearing an electrical charge.

vv. The measure of acid and base strength.

## Fill in the Blank

Fill in the blanks with information from the key terms used in this chapter.

1. An _____ is an ion bearing a negative charge.

2. A _____ is an ion bearing a positive charge.

3. An _____ is an atom bearing an electrical charge.

4. An _____ is a basic substance of matter.

## Abbreviation Review

Write the meaning or definition of the following abbreviations, acronyms, and symbols.

1. ABG _____

2. ADH _____

3. ATP _____

4. BP _____

5. BUN _____

6. $Ca^{++}$ _____

7. CBC _____

8. $Cl^-$ _____

9. $CO_2^-$ _____

10. COOH _____

11. CNS _____

12. $D_5W$ _____

13. dL _____

14. ECF _____

15. GI _____

16. $H^+$ _____

17. $H_2CO_3$ _____

18. $H_2O$ _____

19. HCl _____

20. $HCO_3^-$ _____

21. Hct _____

22. Hgb _____

23. I&O _____

24. ICF _____

25. IV _____

26. $K^+$ _____

27. KCl _____

28. kg _____

29. L _____

30. lb. _____

31. mEq _____

32. mg _____

33. $Mg^{++}$ _____

34. mL _____

35. mm Hg _____

36. MOM _____

37. mOsm/kg _____

38. $Na^+$ _____

39. NaCl _____

40. $NaH_2PO_4$ _____

41. $NaHCO_3$ _____

42. $NaHPO_4$ _____

43. NaOH _____

44. $NH_2$ _____

45. NPO _____

46. $O_2$ _____

47. OH _____

48. $PCO_2$ ($PaCO_2$) _____

49. pH _____

50. $PO_2$ ($PaO_2$) _____

51. $PO_4^-$ _____

52. $SaO_2$ _____

53. TPN _____

54. TPR _____

55. wt _____

## Exercises and Activities

1. Complete the following statements:

   a. Understanding fluid and electrolyte balance is important for the nurse because

   _____

   _____

   b. Homeostasis can be described as

   _____

   _____

   c. The body tries to maintain homeostasis by

   _____

   _____

2. Use the following diagrams to describe the processes of osmosis and diffusion.

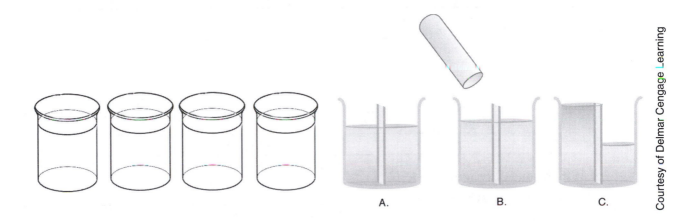

A.          B.          C.

Draw and explain diffusion:                    Draw and explain osmosis:

a. What is hemolysis and how does it occur?

_____

_____

b. How does dialysis work?

_____

_____

3. Why is it important for the body to maintain the acid–base balance?

_____

_____

_____

a. How does each of the body's three main control systems regulate acid–base balance?

The buffer systems: _____

_____

_____

Respiratory regulation: _____

_____

_____

Renal regulation: _____

_____

_____

b. Which control system is fastest? _____
Which control system is slowest? _____

4. List signs of a fluid imbalance that a nurse might observe on physical examination of a client per age group.

| Fluid Volume Excess | Adult | Child |
|---|---|---|
| (1) | | |
| (2) | | |
| (3) | | |
| (4) | | |
| Fluid Volume Deficit | Adult | Child |
| (1) | | |
| (2) | | |
| (3) | | |
| (4) | | |

a. Why is dehydration a common and serious fluid imbalance in an individual?

_____

_____

b. What are the primary nursing goals in dehydration?

_____

_____

c. Explain why 0.9% NaCl could be used for fluid replacement.

_____

_____

d. What would you tell a client about the role that water plays in health?

_____

_____

5. S.B. is a 29-year-old client who arrived at the hospital with multiple trauma following an automobile accident. Because of injury to his lungs, S.B. is now acutely ill. On assessment, the nurse notes that he is showing signs of hypoxemia, including dyspnea, increased respiratory rate, and an increased heart rate. He has been restless since he was admitted, but now appears to be showing some confusion.

a. The nurse determines that S.B. is exhibiting signs of which acid–base imbalance?

_____

_____

b. What changes in laboratory values would you anticipate?

pH _____

$PCO_2$ _____

$HCO_3$ _____

c. Why is a prompt and careful respiratory assessment important for this client?

_____

_____

d. List three actual or risk nursing diagnoses for this client.

(1) _____

(2) _____

(3) _____

e. How does respiratory acidosis differ from metabolic acidosis?

_____

_____

6. Fill in the table.

*Acid Base Review*

|  | Respiratory Acidosis | Respiratory Alkalosis |
|---|---|---|
| pH |  |  |
| PCO$_2$ levels |  |  |
| HCO$_3$ levels |  |  |
|  | Metaboic Acidosis | Metabolic Alkalosis |
| pH |  |  |
| PCO$_2$ levels |  |  |
| HCO$_3$ levels |  |  |

## Self-Assessment Questions

Circle the letter that corresponds to the best answer.

1. The human body can tolerate only very slight changes in
   a. fluid volume.
   b. metabolic rate.
   c. respiratory rate.
   d. blood pH value.

2. If blood pH falls below 7.35, acidosis occurs, which may be characterized by a weak and irregular heartbeat, lower blood pressure, and
   a. a decreased level of consciousness (LOC).
   b. a decreased respiratory rate.
   c. spasmodic muscle contractions.
   d. numbness and tingling in the extremities.

3. A client admitted with dehydration may exhibit signs and symptoms that include dry mucous membranes, decreased tearing, decreased urine output, and
   a. decreased pulse rate.
   b. lower blood pressure.
   c. jugular vein distention.
   d. taut, smooth, shiny, pale skin.

4. The hormones ADH, aldosterone, and renin are important to a client's health status because they
   a. maintain the fluid balance by encouraging the kidneys to retain water.
   b. maintain the acid–base balance by causing the excretion of sodium.
   c. stabilize the normal pH level as part of the buffer systems.
   d. bind with excess hydrogen ions in the blood.

5. A client tells the nurse that he has been taking a lot of antacid tablets and milk in an attempt to control heartburn. The nurse should be aware that this client may be at risk for
   a. gastric acidosis.
   b. metabolic acidosis.
   c. metabolic alkalosis.
   d. compensatory alkalosis.

6. The most common indicator in a client who has fluid volume deficit is
   a. thirst.
   b. weakness.
   c. decreased urination.
   d. increased skin turgor.

7. A client has been advised to take a calcium supplement. To increase her absorption of calcium from the gastrointestinal tract, the nurse explains to the client that she should also consume
   a. vitamin C.
   b. vitamin D.
   c. amino acids.
   d. sports drinks.

8. An example of an isotonic solution is
   a. 0.45% NaCl.
   b. 0.9% NaCl.
   c. 3% NaCl.
   d. 5% dextrose in 0.9% NaCl.

9. A _____ solution would cause crenation.
   a. hypotonic
   b. isotonic
   c. hypertonic
   d. osmotic

10. The client received a crushing injury to the leg when a tree fell on it. With a crush injury, the nurse anticipates which of the following electrolytes will be elevated as a result of the intracellular damage?
    a. Sodium
    b. Bicarbonate
    c. Chloride
    d. Potassium

# Medication Administration and IV Therapy

## Key Terms

Match the following terms with their correct definitions.

___ 1. Absorption

___ 2. Angiocatheter

___ 3. Aspiration

___ 4. Bioavailability

___ 5. Butterfly needle

___ 6. Chemical name

___ 7. Distribution

___ 8. Drug allergy

___ 9. Drug incompatibility

___10. Drug interaction

___11. Drug tolerance

___12. Enteral instillation

___13. Excretion

___14. Extravasation

a. Hypersensitivity to a drug.

b. Time it takes the body to eliminate half of the blood concentration level of the original dose.

c. Device made of a radiopaque silicone catheter and a plastic or stainless steel injection port with a self-sealing silicone-rubber septum.

d. Study of the absorption, distribution, metabolism, and excretion of drugs to determine the relationship between the dose of a drug and the drug's concentration in biological fluids.

e. Physical and chemical processing of a drug by the body.

f. Seepage of foreign substances into the interstitial tissue, causing swelling and discomfort at the IV site.

g. Procedure performed to withdraw fluid that has abnormally collected or to obtain a specimen; also, inhalation of regurgitated gastric contents into the pulmonary system.

h. Medications dispensed and labeled in large quantities for storage in the medication room or nursing unit.

i. Effect one drug can have on another drug.

j. Highly unpredictable response that may be manifested by an overresponse, an underresponse, or an atypical response.

k. System of packaging and labeling each dose of medication by the pharmacy, usually for a 24-hour period.

l. Addition of an intravenous solution to infuse concurrently with another infusion.

m. The highest blood concentration of a single dose until the elimination rate equals the rate of absorption.

n. Passage of a drug from the site of administration into the bloodstream.

___15. Flashback

___16. Flow rate

___17. Generic name

___18. Half-life

___19. Hypervolemia

___20. Idiosyncratic reaction

___21. Implantable port

___22. Infiltration

___23. Intracath

___24. Intradermal

___25. Intramuscular

___26. Intravenous

___27. IV push (bolus)

___28. Metabolism

___29. Onset of action

___30. Parenteral

___31. Patency

___32. Peak plasma level

___33. Pharmacokinetics

___34. Phlebitis

___35. Piggyback

___36. Plateau

___37. Stock supply

___38. Subcutaneous

___39. Toxic effect

___40. Trade (brand) name

___41. Unit dose form

___42. Vesicant

o. Precise description of the drug's composition (chemical formula).

p. Method of administering a large dose of medication in a relatively short time, usually 1 to 30 minutes.

q. Level at which a drug's blood concentration is maintained.

r. Medication that causes blisters and tissue injury when it escapes into surrounding tissue.

s. Increased circulating fluid volume.

t. Administration of drugs through a gastrointestinal tube.

u. Wing-tipped needle.

v. Intracatheter with a metal stylet.

w. Plastic tube for insertion into a vein.

x. Time it takes the body to respond to a drug after administration.

y. Being freely opened.

z. Inflammation of a vein.

aa. Injection into the subcutaneous tissue.

bb. Name assigned by the U.S. Adopted Names Council to the manufacturer that first develops the drug.

cc. Any route other than the oral–gastrointestinal tract.

dd. Injection into the dermis.

ee. Readiness to produce a drug effect.

ff. Undesired chemical or physical reaction between a drug and a solution, between two drugs, or between a drug and the container or tubing.

gg. Volume of fluid to infuse over a set period of time.

hh. Name assigned a drug by the pharmaceutical company.

ii. Elimination of drugs from the body.

jj. Reaction that occurs when the body becomes accustomed to a specific drug and requires larger doses of the drug to produce the desired therapeutic effects.

kk. Movement of drugs from the blood into various body fluids and tissues.

ll. Injection into the muscle.

mm. Injection into a vein.

nn. Reaction that occurs when the body cannot metabolize a drug, causing the drug to accumulate in the blood.

oo. Rushing of blood back into intravenous tubing when a negative pressure is created on the tubing.

pp. The inadvertent IV administration of a vesicant escaping into the surrounding tissue.

## Fill in the Blank

1. The _____ and the _____ are books of drug standards in the United States.

2. The _____, or nonproprietary drug name, is assigned by the U.S. Adopted Names Council. These names are not capitalized.

3. _____ refers to the routes of medication administration that are *not* the oral-gastrointestinal route.

4. The movement of a drug from the administration site into the bloodstream is known as _____.

## Abbreviation Review

Write the meaning or definition of the following abbreviations, acronyms, and symbols.

1. AIDS _____
2. BSA _____
3. c _____
4. cc _____
5. cm _____
6. CVC _____
7. $D_5W$ _____
8. DEA _____
9. dr _____
10. FDA _____
11. fl _____
12. g _____
13. GI _____
14. gr _____
15. gtt _____
16. ID _____
17. IM _____
18. IV _____
19. IVPB _____
20. kg _____
21. KVO _____
22. L _____
23. lb _____
24. ɱ _____
25. MAR _____
26. mcg _____
27. mg _____
28. min _____
29. mL _____

30. NF _____

31. NG _____

32. NPO _____

33. NTG _____

34. oz _____

35. po _____

36. prn _____

37. pt _____

38. PT _____

39. PTT _____

40. qd _____

41. qt _____

42. RBC _____

43. SC/SQ _____

44. tsp _____

45. Tbsp _____

46. USP _____

47. VAD _____

## Exercises and Activities

1. Explain the benefits of each of the following methods of medication administration.

   Buccal _____

   Intramuscular _____

   Intravenous _____

   Oral _____

   Respiratory _____

   Subcutaneous _____

   Sublingual _____

   Topical _____

2. What are the nurse's responsibilities related to giving medications?

   _____

   _____

   _____

   a. What was the impact of the Controlled Substance Act of 1970?

   _____

   _____

   b. List and briefly describe the four properties that determine the action of a drug.

   (1) _____

   (2) _____

   (3) _____

   (4) _____

c. How does the onset of action influence the choice of route for a drug?

_____

_____

d. Why are most medications given orally?

_____

_____

3. What questions will the nurse ask clients about their medication history?

_____

_____

_____

a. If a client states she has an allergic reaction to a particular medication, what information is needed?

_____

_____

b. How can you help prepare a client to take medication at home?

_____

_____

c. List the seven "rights" of medication administration.

(1) _____

(2) _____

(3) _____

(4) _____

(5) _____

(6) _____

(7) _____

d. If you make a medication error, what steps should you take?

_____

_____

e. What actions should the nurse take if the client refuses to take the prescribed medications?

_____

_____

f. How is noncompliance different from refusing to take a dose of medication?

_____

_____

4. Give the equivalent (approximate) for each measurement:

| | | | | | | |
|---|---|---|---|---|---|---|
| 1 gr | = _____ mg | 1 cup | = _____ oz | 1 Tbsp | = _____ mL |
| 1 g | = _____ mg | 1/2 cup | = _____ cc | 1 mL | = _____ minim |
| 1 tsp | = _____ cc | 1 kg | = _____ lb | 5 ft. 8 in. | = _____ cm |
| 1 L | = _____ mL | 1 lb | = _____ kg | 60 kg | = _____ lb |
| 1 oz | = _____ cc | 1 oz | = _____ Tbsp | 0.5 mg | = _____ mcg |
| 0.5 L | = _____ mL | 1 tsp | = _____ gtt | gr 1/200 | = _____ mg |

a. Determine the correct dosage for the following medication orders.

(1) You need to administer Benadryl 50 mg po every six hours as needed for itching. If each capsule is 25 mg, how many capsules will you give? _____ What is the maximum number of mg of Benadryl your client might receive in 24 hours? _____

(2) You need to administer phenobarbital gr 1/2 po. If each tablet is 60 mg, how many tablets will you give? _____

(3) You are giving ampicillin 325 mg IV to an infant. After the medication is reconstituted, it equals 250 mg/mL. How many cc will you give? _____

(4) You are also administering gentamicin 8 mg IM. The vial contains 40 mg/mL. How many cc will you give?_____ What size syringe will you use? _____ What site will you use for this injection? _____

(5) An IV of 1,000 mL D5W is scheduled to infuse at a rate of 125 mL/hr. If you start it at 1300, when will it finish? _____

(6) On the following diagram of a 3 cc syringe, draw a line at 1.6 cc.

Courtesy of Delmar Cengage Learning

b. What is the body surface area for a newborn, 21 in. in height, weighing 9 lb? _____
What is the body surface area for a child 90 cm in height, weighing 14 kg? _____

c. What information is missing from the following medication orders for Mr. J. Client?

(1) *8/31/xx 1130 Tetracycline 250 mg po x 5 days. Dr. B. Smith*

Missing: _____

(2) *9/1/xx Lanoxin 0.125 mg q AM at 0900 Dr. B. Smith*

Missing: _____

5. Using the computerized medication record (Figure 25-3 in your text), answer the following questions.

What is the client's diagnosis? _____

What does "start date" mean? _____

List the medications that L. White gave at 9 A.M. _____

What does QOD indicate on the Lanoxin order? _____

If the client has chest pain, what will you give? _____

When is Reglan ordered to be given? _____

When was the last time Mr. Patient took pain medication? _____

What were the medication and dose given for pain? _____

Where was the injection given? _____

You are caring for this client from 3 P.M. to 11 P.M. List the drug name, dose, and time of all the medications you will be responsible for giving. _____

_____

6. A new nurse is preparing to give medications to several clients on her unit this morning.

   a. Her first client, J.B., is to have 10 units of regular insulin with breakfast. The nurse remembers from class that insulin is given subcutaneously because _____. J.B. tells the nurse that he usually gives himself injections in his thighs when he is at home and asks the nurse to use a different site. Draw on the following diagram the sites the nurse could use for J.B.

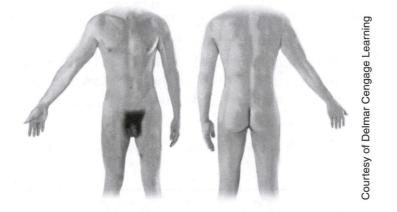

Courtesy of Delmar Cengage Learning

   b. In the next room, the nurse will start one of the two antibiotics due at 8 A.M., IVPB, on A.R. Why will Kim check drug compatibility on the two medications?

   _____

   _____

   Before starting the first antibiotic, the nurse assesses the IV site in A.R.'s right forearm. She recalls that the signs and symptoms of infiltration and phlebitis are

   _____

   _____.

   If the nurse determines that A.R. has phlebitis, she will

   _____

   _____.

   The nurse sets the flow rate for the IV. Because the IV of 1,000 mL is ordered to run for 12 hours, the nurse determines the infusion rate as _____ mL/hr. Because she is not using an infusion pump, she calculates the IV drip rate. The drip factor for this IV tubing is 12 drops/mL. She calculates the IV drip rate as _____ drops per minute. List five actions/interventions that the nurse will include in monitoring this client's IV therapy.

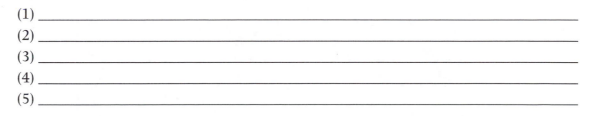

c. Her next client, C.W., is on I&O. After C.W. finishes with her clear liquid breakfast tray, the nurse asks what she had to drink. C.W. says, "I had a cup of bouillon, half a cup of juice, and an ounce of water with a pain pill earlier." The nurse writes down _____ mL as C.W.'s fluid intake for breakfast.

d. N.P., a client the nurse remembers from a previous admission, is waiting for her in the next room. He is scheduled to have an IM injection of iron dextran (Imferon) this morning. She will inject this drug deeply into the _____ site using the Z-track method. To use the Z-track method, the nurse will _____

_____.

e. Depending on lab work this morning, S.Z., the nurse's last client, may need to have packed RBCs administered again today. What items will the nurse include in her initial assessment and preparation for S.Z. to receive blood products? _____

_____.

7. Identify the needle gauge, length, and angle of entry that are used in the following types of injections.

| Injection Type | Needle Gauge | Needle Length | Angle of Entry |
| --- | --- | --- | --- |
| Intradermal | | | |
| Subcutaneous | | | |
| Insulin | | | |
| Intramuscular | | | |

a. Name the muscles that the nurse would give an injection in at the following sites.
   (1) Upper arm _____
   (2) Thigh _____
   (3) Buttocks _____
   (4) Hip _____

b. The client is receiving a transfusion of packed red blood cells for anemia. The nurse needs to observe for signs of a trasnsfusion reaction. List the symptoms.

_____

_____

## Self-Assessment Questions

Circle the letter that corresponds to the best answer for each question.

1. Parenteral drugs are administered by all except which of the following routes?
   a. Intraspinal
   b. Sublingual
   c. Intradermal
   d. Subcutaneous

2. A client is considered to be noncompliant with his medication. The nurse should first determine
   a. whether the client really needs the medicine.
   b. how to get the client to take the medication.
   c. why the client is not taking the drug as prescribed.
   d. whether there is a similar drug the client can take instead.

3. Drug actions are dependent on their absorption, distribution, metabolism, and
   a. excretion.
   b. utilization.
   c. bioavailability.
   d. administration.

4. The nurse caring for a new client notes during the assessment that he has difficulty swallowing. A medication was ordered for this client in tablet form. To avoid aspiration, the nurse will
   a. give the medication by injection.
   b. ask the physician to change the order.
   c. crush the tablet and mix it with water or juice.
   d. find a similar medication that is easier to swallow.

5. The nurse is preparing to give a medication to the client, who states, "This is a new pill. Why are you giving this to me?" The nurse should first
   a. check the medication order again.
   b. tell the client why she needs the medication.
   c. hold the medication until the physician comes in the next morning.
   d. explain why it is important to take the medications prescribed by the doctor.

6. A nurse is assessing the IV site on a client and notes the presence of swelling and cool, pale skin. The nurse understands that these are signs of
   a. phlebitis.
   b. infiltration.
   c. catheter sepsis.
   d. rapid IV infusion.

7. Anabolic steroids are a schedule ___ drug.
   a. I
   b. II
   c. III
   d. IV

8. Diazepam is a schedule ___ drug.
   a. I
   b. II
   c. III
   d. IV

9. A severe life-threatening reaction to a drug is called
   a. urticaria.
   b. anaphylaxis.
   c. tolerance.
   d. a toxic effect.

10. A nurse on your unit has an emergency situation occurring and asks you to administer medications already prepared. You should
   a. give the medications.
   b. help with the emergency.
   c. prepare and administer the medications yourself.
   d. refuse and leave the medications in the medication room.

# Assessment

## Chapter 26

## Key Terms

Match the following terms with their correct definitions.

___ 1. Adventitious breath sound

___ 2. Affect

___ 3. Auscultation

___ 4. Borborygmi

___ 5. Bradycardia

___ 6. Bradypnea

___ 7. Bronchial sound

___ 8. Bronchovesicular sound

___ 9. Crackles

___10. Cyanosis

___11. Dyspnea

___12. Eupnea

___13. Health history

___14. Hyperventilation

a. High-pitched, loud, rushing sounds produced by the movement of gas in the liquid contents of the intestine.

b. Physical examination technique that uses the sense of touch to assess texture, temperature, moisture, organ location and size, vibrations and pulsations, swelling, masses, and tenderness.

c. High-pitched, harsh sound heard on inspiration when the trachea or larynx is obstructed.

d. Bluish or dark purple discoloration of the lips, skin, or nail beds.

e. Indirect measurement of cardiac output obtained by counting the number of peripheral pulse waves over a pulse point.

f. Low-pitched grating sound on inhalation and exhalation.

g. Respiratory rate greater than 24 beats per minute.

h. Abnormal, low-pitched breath sound, louder on exhalation.

i. Abnormal breath sound.

j. Abnormal breath sound that resembles a popping sound, heard in inhalation and exhalation, not cleared by coughing.

k. Review of the client's functional health patterns prior to the current contact with a health care agency.

l. Physical examination technique that involves listening to sounds in the body that are created by movement of air or fluid.

m. Heart rate less than 60 beats per minute in an adult.

n. Physical examination technique that uses short, tapping strokes on the surface of the skin to create vibrations of underlying organs.

___15. Hypoventilation

o. Condition in which the apical pulse rate is greater than the radial pulse rate.

___16. Inspection

p. Regularity of the heartbeat.

___17. Orthostatic hypotension

q. Chart containing various-sized letters with standardized numbers at the end of each line of letters.

___18. Palpation

r. Brief account of any recent signs or symptoms related to any body system.

___19. Percussion

s. Medium-pitched and blowing sounds heard equally on inspiration and expiration from air moving through the large airways.

___20. Pleural friction rub

t. Easy respirations with a rate of breaths per minute that is age appropriate.

___21. Pulse amplitude

u. Outward expression of mood or emotions.

___22. Pulse deficit

v. Respiratory rate of 10 or fewer breaths per minute.

___23. Pulse rate

w. Physical examination technique that involves thorough visual observation.

___24. Pulse rhythm

x. Heart rate in excess of 100 beats per minute in an adult.

___25. Review of systems

y. Abnormal breath sound, high pitched and whistlelike in nature, during inhalation and exhalation.

___26. Sibilant wheeze

z. Breathing characterized by shallow respirations.

___27. Snellen chart

aa. Soft, breezy, low-pitched sound heard longer on inspiration than expiration that results from air moving through the smaller airways over the lung periphery, with the exception of the scapular area.

___28. Sonorous wheeze

bb. Measurement of the strength or force exerted by the ejected blood against the arterial wall with each contraction.

___29. Stridor

cc. Difficulty breathing as observed by labored or forced respirations through the use of accessory muscles in the chest and neck.

___30. Tachycardia

dd. Loud, tubular, hollow-sounding breath sound normally heard over the sternum.

___31. Tachypnea

ee. Significant decrease in blood pressure that results with dizziness or lightheadedness when a person moves from a lying or sitting (supine) position to a standing position.

___32. Vesicular sound

ff. Breathing characterized by deep, rapid respirations.

## Abbreviation Review

Write the meaning or definition of the following abbreviations, acronyms, and symbols.

1. BP _____

2. cm _____

3. LLQ _____

4. LOC _____

5. LUQ _____

6. P _____

7. PERRLA _____

8. R _____

9. RLQ _____

10. ROS _____

11. RUQ _____

12. T _____

## Exercises and Activities

1. Personal data including name, address, birth date, and gender are known as _____ information.

2. In addition to physical assessment, identify four other sources of objective data.

   a._____

   b._____

   c._____

   d._____

3. What does *light accommodation* stand for in assessing for PERRLA?

   _____

4. What is the frequency of bowel sounds if they are normally active?

   _____

5. What are the purposes of the health history and physical assessment?

   _____

   _____

   _____

   a.  What findings might indicate that a client has been abused?

   _____

   _____

6. In which section of the health history would each of the following items be found?

   a. Completed hepatitis immunization _____

   b. Smokes one pack of cigarettes a day _____

   c. Last Pap test 6 months ago _____

   d. Experiencing stress from a new job _____

   e. Client rates his health as an 8 on a scale of 1 to 10 _____

   f.  Sister and maternal grandmother have high blood pressure _____

   g. Develops a rash with penicillin _____

    h. Began having severe stomach pain 1 hour ago _____

    i. Sleeps 7 hours a night, feels rested _____

    j. Thyroidectomy at age 24 _____

    k. Takes acetaminophen 650 mg every 4 hours PRN for headache _____

    l. Chickenpox at age 5, no sequelae _____

7. Write at least two interventions that might be helpful for assessing each of the following:

    An elderly client: _____
_____

    A client who is hearing impaired: _____
_____

    A client who is dyspneic: _____
_____

    A client who does not speak English: _____
_____

    A client who is in pain: _____
_____

8. What items are included in the assessment of vital signs?

    a. Give normal findings for T-P-R and BP.
_____
_____
_____

    b. Why are vital signs an important part of an assessment?
_____
_____

    c. What factors can affect an individual's temperature, pulse, respirations, and blood pressure?
_____
_____

    d. Convert the following temperatures:

    97.7°F = _____ °C    38°C = _____ °F
    101°F = _____ °C    39°C = _____ °F

    e. Explain the following terms:
      (1) Bradycardia _____
      (2) Bradypnea _____
      (3) Dyspnea _____
      (4) Eupnea _____
      (5) Hypoventilation _____

(6) Hyperventilation _____

(7) Tachycardia _____

(8) Tachypnea _____

f.  Label and draw a line to each of the pulse points on the figure.

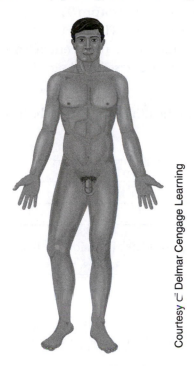

g.  Draw an X over each area on this diagram where you would auscultate the lungs. Draw an arrow to show where you would assess the apical pulse.

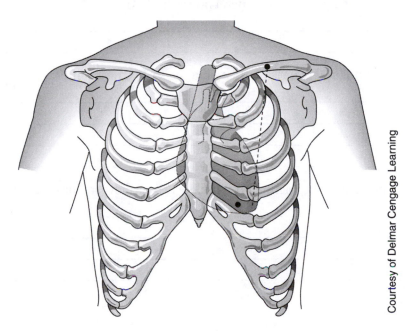

h. Write a brief description of normal findings for a respiratory assessment on a client.

_____

_____

9. D.M. is a 71-year-old client with a history of cigarette smoking, obesity, hypertension, and diabetes mellitus. Vital signs are temperature 97.9°F, pulse 88, respirations 20, blood pressure 158/92, and a weight today of 213 lb. He is now exhibiting signs and symptoms of peripheral vascular disease, a complication of poorly controlled diabetes. During your assessment of the lower extremities, you note decreased leg hair, skin that is cool to touch, with some loss of sensation.

a. What information from his health history might be helpful in planning nursing interventions and teaching for D.M.?

_____

_____

_____

_____

b. Write three questions you could ask D.M. for the ROS for his legs.

(1) _____

(2) _____

(3) _____

c. What other information could you obtain during your physical examination of the legs?

_____

_____

d. Where will you palpate the peripheral pulses for D.M.?

_____

_____

e. Write two actual and two risk nursing diagnoses for this client.

(1) _____

(2) _____

(3) _____

(4) _____

f. What elements will you include to complete the cardiovascular assessment of this client?

_____

_____

_____

_____

## Self-Assessment Questions

Circle the letter that corresponds to the best answer.

1. The nurse is performing percussion on the client's abdomen. If the assessment findings are normal, the nurse would note
   a. stridor.
   b. tympany.
   c. resonance.
   d. hyperresonance.

2. The nurse is preparing to do a physical assessment on an elderly client with difficulty breathing. Which position will the nurse use for respiratory assessment?
   a. Sims
   b. Supine
   c. Sitting
   d. Dorsal recumbent

3. An abdominal assessment finding that the nurse will report to a supervisor is
   a. positive borborygmi.
   b. audible peristalsis on auscultation.
   c. separation of the rectus abdominis muscle.
   d. finding abdominal organs with light palpation.

4. A nurse is performing a head and neck assessment on the client. To assess for visual acuity, the nurse will use
   a. a Snellen chart.
   b. direct light reflex.
   c. tangential lighting.
   d. an ophthalmoscope.

5. To accurately assess the apical pulse of a client, the nurse will
   a. palpate the brachial artery and count for 30 seconds.
   b. locate the left carotid artery and palpate gently for 1 minute.
   c. locate the fifth intercostal space, midclavicular line, and listen for 60 seconds.
   d. place the stethoscope on the left of the sternum and listen for 30 seconds.

6. The nurse is auscultating the lungs of a client with a respiratory illness. The breath sounds over the periphery of the lungs are normally described as
   a. resonant.
   b. vesicular.
   c. bronchial.
   d. hyperresonant.

7. A technique requiring significant expertise and instructor supervision is
   a. light palpation.
   b. auscultation.
   c. visual observation.
   d. deep palpation.

8. The best position for assessment of the abdomen is
    a. sitting.
    b. dorsal recumbent.
    c. supine.
    d. Sims'.

9. The _____ position is indicated for the assessment of the lungs of a client with cardiopulmonary alterations.
    a. sitting
    b. dorsal recumbent
    c. supine
    d. Sims'

10. All are life-cycle considerations for an elderly client except
    a. senses that are less acute.
    b. increased awareness to pain.
    c. decreased height.
    d. slowed respirations.

# Pain Management

## Key Terms

Match the following terms with their correct definitions.

___ 1. Acupuncture

___ 2. Acute pain

___ 3. Adjuvant medication

___ 4. Afferent pain pathway

___ 5. Analgesia

___ 6. Analgesic

___ 7. Ceiling effect

___ 8. Chronic acute pain

___ 9. Chronic nonmalignant pain

___10. Chronic pain

___11. Colic

___12. Cryotherapy

a. Discomfort identified by sudden onset and relatively short duration, mild to severe intensity, and a steady decrease in intensity over several days or weeks.

b. Discomfort that occurs almost daily, has been present for at least 6 months, and ranges in intensity from mild to severe; also known as chronic benign pain.

c. Descending spinal cord pathway that transmits sensory impulses from the brain.

d. Neuropathic pain that occurs after amputation with pain sensations referred to an area in the missing portion of the limb.

e. Unpleasant sensory and emotional experience associated with actual or potential tissue damage or described in terms of such.

f. Compound that blocks opioid effects on one receptor type while producing opioid effects on a second receptor type.

g. Drug used to enhance the analgesic efficacy of opioids, treat concurrent symptoms that exacerbate pain, and provide independent analgesia for specific types of pain.

h. Use of cold applications to reduce swelling.

i. Analgesics administered via a catheter that terminates in the epidural space.

j. Technique of focusing attention on stimuli other than pain.

k. State of heightened awareness and focused concentration.

l. Discomfort from the internal organs that is felt in another area of the body.

___13. Cutaneous pain

___14. Distraction

___15. Efferent pain pathway

___16. Endorphins

___17. Epidural analgesia

___18. Gate control pain theory

___19. Hypnosis

___20. Intrathecal analgesia

___21. Ischemic pain

___22. Mixed agonist-antagonist

___23. Modulation

___24. Myofascial pain syndromes

___25. Neuralgia

___26. Nociceptor

___27. Noxious stimulus

___28. Pain

___29. Pain threshold

___30. Pain tolerance

___31. Patient-controlled analgesia

___32. Perception

m. Stress management strategy in which muscles are alternately tensed and relaxed.

n. Underlying pathology that causes pain.

o. Central nervous system pathway that selectively inhibits pain transmission by sending signals back down to the dorsal horn of the spinal cord.

p. Paroxysmal pain that extends along the course of one or more nerves.

q. Noxious stimulus that triggers electrical activity in the endings of afferent nerve fibers (nociceptors).

r. Process of applying a low-voltage electrical current to the skin through cutaneous electrodes.

s. Phenomenon of requiring larger and larger doses of an analgesic to achieve the same level of pain relief.

t. Discomfort resulting when the blood supply of an area is restricted or cut off completely.

u. Level of intensity at which pain becomes appreciable or perceptible.

v. Device that allows the client to control the delivery of intravenous or subcutaneous pain medication in a safe, effective manner through a programmable pump.

w. Discomfort marked by repetitive painful episodes that may recur over a prolonged period or throughout a client's lifetime.

x. Technique of monitoring negative thoughts and replacing them with positive ones.

y. Discomfort caused by stimulation of the cutaneous nerve endings in the skin.

z. Group of opiate-like substances produced naturally by the brain; these substances raise the pain threshold, produce sedation and euphoria, and promote a sense of well-being.

aa. Pain relief without producing anesthesia.

bb. Ascending spinal cord.

cc. Administration of analgesics into the subarachnoid space.

dd. Receptive neuron for painful sensations.

ee. Nonlocalized discomfort originating in tendons, ligaments, and nerves.

ff. Level of intensity or duration of pain that a person is willing to endure.

___33. Phantom limb pain

gg. Discomfort generally identified as long term (lasting 6 months or longer) that is persistent, nearly constant, or recurrent and that produces significant negative changes in a person's life.

___34. Progressive muscle relaxation

hh. Insertion of small needles into the skin at selected (hoku) sites.

___35. Recurrent acute pain

ii. Substance that relieves pain.

___36. Referred pain

jj. Condition of acute abdominal pain.

___37. Reframing

kk. Discomfort that occurs almost daily over a long period, has the potential for lasting months or years, and has a high probability of ending; also known as progressive pain.

___38. Relaxation technique

ll. Theory that proposes that the cognitive, sensory, emotional, and physiological components of the body can act together to block an individual's perception of pain.

___39. Somatic pain

mm. Group of muscle disorders characterized by pain, muscle spasm, tenderness, stiffness, and limited motion.

___40. Tolerance

nn. Process whereby the pain impulse travels from the receiving nociceptors to the spinal cord.

41 Transcutaneous electrical nerve stimulation

oo Method used to decrease anxiety and muscle tension,

___42. Transduction

pp. Discomfort felt in the internal organs.

___43. Transmission

qq. Ability to experience, recognize, organize, and interpret sensory stimuli.

___44. Visceral pain

rr. Medication dosage beyond which no further analgesia occurs.

## Abbreviation Review

Write the meaning or definition of the following abbreviations, acronyms, and symbols.

1. APS _____

2. AHCPR _____

3. ATC _____

4. EMLA _____

5. IASP _____

6. MRI _____

7. NPO _____

8. NSAID _____

9. PCA _____

10. PRN _____

11. TAC _____

12. TENS _____

13. TMJ _____

14. VAS _____

15. WHO _____

## Exercises and Activities

1. In what ways is the role of the nurse important in pain relief?

_____

_____

_____

_____

   a. What is the importance of pain control to an individual's health?

   _____

   _____

   _____

   _____

   b. When is pain deemed chronic?

   _____

   _____

   _____

   _____

   c. How can pain be a diagnostic tool?

   _____

   _____

   _____

   _____

2. Draw and label the pain pathway from the stimulus to the muscle response.

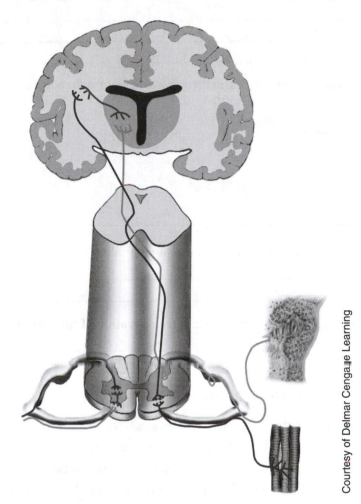

Courtesy of Delmar Cengage Learning

a. How does each of the following factors affect how an individual experiences pain?

Age: _____

_____

Previous experiences with pain: _____

_____

Cultural norms: _____

_____

b. Briefly describe the three general principles of pain management.

_____

_____

3. How does the nurse determine the amount of pain a client is experiencing?

_____

_____

_____

a. Compare and give examples for the three categories of pain control interventions.

|  | Examples | Advantages | Disadvantages |
|---|---|---|---|
| Pharmacological |  |  |  |
| Noninvasive |  |  |  |
| Invasive |  |  |  |

b. How do nonopioid analgesics differ from opioid analgesics?

_____

_____

c. What are the nurse's responsibilities in administration of analgesics?

_____

_____

4. A client gives the following description of a headache:

"About 2 hours ago I started getting this awful headache right in the back of my head, just above my neck. I've had plenty of headaches before, but this one just came on with no warning, and now it feels like someone is pounding a hammer inside my head. I started feeling sick to my stomach and even vomited a couple of times, but it didn't help. All I had at home to take for the headache was some mild pain medicine, but it didn't even touch the pain. Since my mother died a couple of years ago from a stroke, every headache I get really worries me."

a. What subjective and objective information would be helpful to assess this client's level of pain?

_____

_____

b. For a complete description of the pain, list at least five specific questions you will ask this client.

(1) _____

(2) _____

(3) _____

(4) _____

(5) _____

c. What terms might clients use to describe the quality of their pain?

_____

_____

d.  Give an example of a nursing diagnosis for this client.

_____

_____

e.  State the goal for the client using the above nursing diagnosis.

_____

_____

5.  F.L. is a 34-year-old client who had an amputation of her right leg below the knee as a result of extensive trauma 3 years ago. Since then, she has experienced chronic neuropathic pain ranging from mild to moderate. With a prosthesis, she is able to care for her family and do housework, but she has difficulty sitting for extended periods of time or walking long distances. F.L. has tried several types of pain medication over the past year but states that the ones that give enough relief make her feel too sleepy.

a.  What type of pain is F.L. experiencing?

_____

_____

b.  List five ways in which the pain F.L. is experiencing differs from acute pain.

(1) _____

(2) _____

(3) _____

(4) _____

(5) _____

c.  Does this client's pain serve as a protective mechanism?

_____

_____

d.  F.L. says that she would like to try something to help ease her pain besides just medication. Suggest two interventions and explain your rationale.

(1) _____

_____

_____

(2) _____

_____

_____

e.  Why will she need ongoing pain assessments?

_____

_____

_____

_____

## Self-Assessment Questions

Circle the letter that corresponds to the best answer.

1. To reverse respiratory depression in a client receiving Duramorph, the nurse would administer
   a. naloxone.
   b. an amphetamine.
   c. an opioid agonist.
   d. a neurolytic agent.
2. The nurse is assessing a client's level and intensity of pain 2 days postsurgery. The most effective way for the nurse to determine the client's pain level is to
   a. evaluate the amount of pain medication taken.
   b. ask the client to describe her perception of the pain.
   c. note the facial expressions and the presence of guarding.
   d. assess the client's mobility and level of self-care activities.

3. As part of a comprehensive pain management plan, noninvasive interventions may include relaxation techniques, guided imagery, distraction, and
   a. radiation.
   b. cryotherapy.
   c. nerve blocks.
   d. nonopioid analgesia.

4. The primary advantage of using PCA is that it
   a. has fewer systemic side effects.
   b. can be used in the home setting.
   c. gives clients greater control over their pain.
   d. uses lower doses of medication to achieve pain relief.

5. A nurse is caring for a client who continues to experience neck and back pain following an automobile accident 1 year ago. Because of the chronic pain, this client is most likely to
   a. use analgesic medication effectively.
   b. display signs that resemble those of anxiety.
   c. exhibit the same behaviors as a client in acute pain.
   d. benefit from nonpharmacological pain relief methods.

6. Twisting an ankle results in
   a. cutaneous pain.
   b. somatic pain.
   c. visceral pain.
   d. referred pain.

7. Signs of chronic pain include
   a. loss of libido and weight.
   b. localized pain and normal vital signs.
   c. guarding and normal pupils.
   d. diaphoresis and fatigue.

8. Myocardial infarction may cause
   a. hormone changes.
   b. colic.
   c. ischemic pain.
   d. myofascial pain.

9. Which side effect of opioid analgesics requires immediate intervention?
   a. Nausea
   b. Constipation
   c. Pruritis
   d. Respiratory depression

10. A noninvasive intervention for pain that uses features of both relaxation and distraction is called
    a. guided imagery.
    b. biofeedback.
    c. reframing.
    d. cognitive-behavioral.

# Diagnostic Tests

## Key Terms

Match the following terms with their correct definitions.

___ 1. Agglutination

___ 2. Agglutinin

___ 3. Agglutinogen

___ 4. Analyte

___ 5. Aneurysm

___ 6. Angiography

___ 7. Antibody

___ 8. Antigen

___ 9. Arteriography

___10. Ascites

___11. Aspiration

___12. Bacteremia

___13. Barium

___14. Biopsy

___15. Central line

___16. Computed tomography

a. Visualization of the vascular structures through the use of fluoroscopy with a contrast medium.

b. Globular protein that is produced in the body and catalyzes chemical reactions within the cells by promoting the oxidative reactions and synthesis of various chemicals.

c. Blood in the urine.

d. Chalky-white contrast medium

e. Venous catheter inserted into the superior vena cava through the subclavian or internal or external jugular vein.

f. Use of high-frequency sound waves to visualize deep body structures; also called an echogram.

g. Study of x-rays or gamma ray–exposed film through the action of ionizing radiation.

h. Diminished production of urine.

i. Minimally depressed level of consciousness during which the client retains the ability to maintain a continuously patent airway and to respond appropriately to physical stimulation or verbal commands.

j. Graphic recording of the heart's electrical activity.

k. Any antigenic substance that causes agglutination by the production of agglutinin.

l. Clumping together of red blood cells.

m. Immunoglobulin produced by the body in response to bacteria, viruses, or other antigenic substances.

n. Substance, usually a protein, that causes the formation of an antibody and reacts specifically with that antibody.

o. Excision of a small amount of tissue.

p. Product of incomplete fat metabolism.

___17. Conscious sedation

q. Aspiration of cerebrospinal fluid from the subarachnoid space.

___18. Contrast medium

r. Process of urine elimination.

___19. Culture

s. Instrument that converts electrical energy to sound waves.

___20. Cytology

t. Susceptibility of a pathogen to an antibiotic.

___21. Electrocardiogram

u. Smear method of examining stained exfoliative cells.

___22. Electroencephalogram

v. Individual who performs venipuncture.

___23. Electrolyte

w. Radiopaque substance that facilitates roentgen (x-ray) imaging of the body's internal structures.

___24. Endoscopy

x. Specific kind of antibody whose interaction with antigens manifests as agglutination.

___25. Enzyme

y. Procedure performed to withdraw fluid that has abnormally collected or to obtain a specimen.

___26. Fluoroscopy

z. Tissue death as the result of disease or injury.

___27. Hematuria

aa. Accessing body tissues, organs, or cavities through some type of instrumentation procedure.

___28. Invasive

bb. Colorless derivative of bilirubin formed by the normal bacterial action of intestinal flora on bilirubin.

___29. Ketone

cc. Alert and with vital signs within the client's normal range.

___30. Lipoprotein

dd. Aspiration of fluid from the abdominal cavity.

___31. Lumbar puncture

ee. Blood in the stool that can be detected only via a microscope or chemical means.

___32. Magnetic resonance imaging

ff. Radiologic scanning of the body with x-ray beams and radiation detectors that transmit data to a computer, which in turn transcribes the data into quantitative measurement and multidimensional images of the internal structures.

___33. Necrosis

gg. Descriptor for procedure wherein the body is not entered with any type of instrument.

___34. Noninvasive

hh. Port that has been implanted under the skin with a catheter inserted into the superior vena cava or right atrium through the subclavian or internal jugular veins.

___35. Occult blood

ii. Immediate, serial images of the body's structure or function.

___36. Oliguria

jj. Abnormal accumulation of fluid in the abdomen.

___37. Papanicolaou test

kk. Weakness in the wall of a blood vessel.

___38. Paracentesis

ll. Growing of microorganisms to identify a pathogen.

___39. Phlebotomist

mm. Graphic recording of the brain's electrical activity.

____40. Pneumothorax

____41. Port-a-Cath

____42. Radiography

____43. Sensitivity

____44. Stable

____45. Stress test

____46. Thoracentesis

____47. Transducer

____48. Trocar

____49. Type and cross-match

____50. Ultrasound

____51. Urobilinogen

____52. Venipuncture

____53. Void

nn. Sharply pointed surgical instrument contained in a cannula.

oo. Visualization of a body organ or cavity through a scope.

pp. Puncturing of a vein with a needle to aspirate blood.

qq. Study of cells.

rr. Blood lipid bound to protein.

ss. Condition of bacteria in the blood.

tt. Substance that is measured.

uu. Substance that, when in solution, separates into ions and conducts electricity.

vv. Radiographic study of the vascular system following the injection of a radiopaque dye through a catheter.

ww. Condition wherein air or gas accumulates in the pleural space, causing the lungs to collapse.

xx. Measure of a client's cardiovascular response to exercise tolerance.

yy. Laboratory test that identifies the client's blood type (e.g., A or B) and determines the compatibility of the blood between potential donor and recipient.

zz. Aspiration of fluids from the pleural cavity.

aaa. Imaging technique that uses radio waves and a strong magnetic field to make continuous cross-sectional images of the body.

## Abbreviation Review

Write the meaning or definition of the following abbreviations and symbols.

1. ABG _____

2. C&S _____

3. CSF _____

4. CT _____

5. ECG (EKG) _____

6. EEG _____

7. IVP _____

8. $PaCO_2$ _____

9. $PaO_2$ _____

10. RBC _____

11. WBC _____

## Exercises and Activities

1. Describe the role of the nurse in preparing a client for diagnostic procedures.

   _____

   _____

   _____

   a. What teaching will the nurse do with the client?

   _____

   _____

   b. Explain the importance of informed consent for invasive procedures.

   _____

   _____

2. What is the role of the nurse during invasive diagnostic procedures?

   _____

   _____

   _____

   a. How can the nurse help the client to be more relaxed?

   _____

   _____

   b. List ways to maintain safety for the nurse and the client during the procedure.

   _____

   _____

3. Identify the purpose of each of these common blood tests and list normal values.

|  | *Normal Values* | *Purpose* |
|---|---|---|
| WBC |  |  |
| Hemoglobin (Hgb) |  |  |
| Hematocrit (Hct) |  |  |
| ABG analysis |  |  |
| $Na^+$ |  |  |
| $K^+$ |  |  |
| Fasting blood sugar (FBS) |  |  |
| Glucose tolerance test (GTT) |  |  |
| Blood urea nitrogen (BUN) |  |  |
| Cholesterol (lipid profile) |  |  |

4. What documentation is the nurse responsible for after diagnostic procedures?

_____

_____

_____

5. For each of the following diagnostic procedures, briefly describe the purpose of the test, any special preparation for the client, and nursing assistance or interventions during the procedure.

|  | *Purpose* | *Preparation* | *Assistance* |
|---|---|---|---|
| Paracentesis |  |  |  |
| Pap smear |  |  |  |
| Cardiac catheterization |  |  |  |
| Thoracentesis |  |  |  |
| Magnetic resonance imaging (MRI) |  |  |  |

6. B.P., a normally active 14-year-old, was brought in by his parents following the sudden onset of a severe headache, nausea, and vomiting. On assessment he appears somewhat irritable and displays stiffness in his neck. His temperature and pulse rate are increased, and he is breathing rapidly. The physician has ordered a lumbar puncture to rule out meningitis. B.P. seems frightened, and the parents are extremely anxious. They insist on staying in the room with their son during the procedure.

a. How does the nurse explain this procedure to B.P.?

_____

_____

b. What preparation is necessary?

_____

_____

c. What position should B.P. assume?

_____

_____

d. How does the nurse assist the physician and B.P. during the procedure?

_____

_____

e. How can the nurse help B.P.'s parents during the procedure?

_____

_____

_____

_____

7. The physician suspects that K.T. has colon cancer. The physician has ordered the following diagnostic tests: Hgb, Hct, CEA, FOBT, abdominal ultrasound, and abdominal CT.

a. K.T. wants to know why blood is being drawn and what is the doctor hoping to find. How should the nurse respond?

_____

_____

_____

b. List the normal laboratory values for:
   (1) Hgb _____
   (2) Hct _____
   (3) CEA _____

c. The nurse instructs K.T. regarding the guiaic test ordered.
   (1) What drugs could affect the results of this test?

   _____

   (2) Why should red meat be avoided in the diet for at least three days prior to this test?

   _____

d. K.T. asks if his bladder needs to be full for the abdominal ultrasound. What should the nurse tell K.T. about an ultrasound exam?

_____

_____

e. The abdominal CT requires the use of contrast media. What safety measures should the nurse take regarding K.T.?

_____

_____

f. K.T. has **K**nowledge Deficit related to diagnostic testing listed as one of his problems on the nursing care plan. What interventions can the nurse take to help K.T.?

_____

_____

## Self-Assessment Questions

Circle the letter that corresponds to the best answer.

1. A nurse is caring for a client who is having an IVP. To monitor the client, the nurse should be aware that the most serious hazard of an allergic reaction to the dye is
   a. oliguria.
   b. urticaria.
   c. respiratory distress.
   d. low blood pressure.

2. A practitioner has ordered a urine sample for a creatinine clearance test. The most appropriate method to collect this is from a
   a. timed sample.
   b. sterile specimen.
   c. random collection.
   d. clean-voided specimen.

3. A nurse is caring for a client who has experienced a bronchoscopy. Following this procedure, it is important for the nurse to
   a. observe the client for signs of tachycardia.
   b. withhold fluids until the gag reflex returns.
   c. advise the client that he may experience dysphagia.
   d. place the client in a high Fowler's position to minimize coughing.

4. The nurse is aware that the most serious complication of thoracentesis is
   a. dyspnea.
   b. infection.
   c. dysrhythmia.
   d. pneumothorax.

5. A client is recovering after having a cardiac catheterization. Following this procedure, it is important for the client to
   a. maintain a side-lying position with the knees bent.
   b. limit fluid intake for several hours until the medication has worn off.
   c. keep the extremity in which the catheter was placed straight and immobile.
   d. collect urine for 24 hours for proper disposal related to the use of radiographic dyes.

6. The nurse correctly describes conscious sedation to the client as
   a. a state of relaxation using biofeedback techniques.
   b. anesthesia delivered by a nurse working in an "expanded role."
   c. a state in which the client is awake and aware but unable to move.
   d. a depressed level of consciousness in which the client can breathe on his own.

7. Immunoglobulins produced by the body in response to bacteria are called
   a. antigens.
   b. antibodies.
   c. agglutinogens.
   d. agglutinins.

8. In an allergic reaction, you would expect to find an increase in _____ when checking the differential count.
   a. neutrophils
   b. eosinophils
   c. lymphocytes
   d. monocytes

9. Which urine test does *not* measure adrenal cortex function?
   a. 17-Hydroxycorticosteroids
   b. Vanillylmandelic acid
   c. Aldosterone assay
   d. Bence Jones protein

10. Which radiologic study can be performed on a client who has an allergy to shellfish?
    a. Cardiac catheterization
    b. Adrenal angiography
    c. Barium enema
    d. Intravenous pyelogram

# Basic Procedures

## Key Terms

Match the following terms with their correct definitions.

___ 1. Antipyretic

___ 2. Antiseptic handwash

___ 3. Antiseptic hand rub

___ 4. Apnea

___ 5. Caries

___ 6. Doppler

___ 7. Gingivitis

___ 8. Halitosis

___ 9. Hand hygiene

___10. Logrolling

___11. Pyrexia

___12. Stomatitis

___13. Surgical hand antisepsis

a. A device used when the pulse cannot be detected by palpation.

b. Bad breath.

c. Cessation of breathing for several seconds.

d. Dental cavities.

e. Fever-reducing medication.

f. Inflammation of the gums.

g. Inflammation of the oral mucosa.

h. Temperature above the normal range.

i. The rubbing together of all surfaces and crevices of the hands using plain soap and water.

j. Turning the client as one unit, keeping the head, neck, hip, and back in alignment.

k. Using an alcohol-based rub to cleanse hands.

l. Using antiseptic handwash or antiseptic hand rub preoperatively by surgical personnel to eliminate transient and reduce resident hand flora.

m. Using antimicrobial substances and water to cleanse hands.

## Abbreviation Review

Write the meaning or definition of the following abbreviations and acronyms.

1. ABCD _____

2. AED _____

3. CDC _____

4. CPR _____

5. EMS _____

6. I&O _____

    7. PMI _____

    8. PROM _____

    9. ROM _____

  10. VRE _____

## Exercises and Activities

1. What are the three essential elements to hand hygiene?

    (1) _____

    (2) _____

    (3) _____

2. List the conditions or times in which hand hygiene should be completed.

    _____

    _____

    _____

    _____

    _____

3. Explain why the hospitalized client is at increased risk for a health care acquired infection.

    _____

    _____

    _____

4. Identify five items used by health care workers to protect themselves from exposure to potentially hazardous body fluids. Include an explanation of when these items are used.

    (1) _____

    (2) _____

    (3) _____

    (4) _____

    (5) _____

5. Describe the correct position/location for each pulse point.

    a. Temporal _____

    b. Carotid _____

    c. Apical _____

    d. Brachial _____

    e. Radial _____

    f. Ulnar _____

    g. Femorai _____

    h. Popliteal _____

    i. Posterior tibial _____

    j. Pedal/dorsal pedal _____

6. What is a nosocomial infection? What are its prevention measures?

_____
_____
_____
_____

7. Describe the anatomical landmarks used when assessing an apical pulse.

_____
_____
_____

8. Explain the five phases of Karotkoff sounds when taking a blood pressure.
   (1) _____
   (2) _____
   (3) _____
   (4) _____
   (5) _____

9. The client is short of breath. The nurse obtains a pulse oximeter reading. The client asks how an oximeter works. How would the nurse explain this to the client?

_____
_____
_____

10. Correct body mechanics are essential in order to avoid _____

_____
_____

11. What is PROM? What is the benefit of PROM? Describe the technique.

_____
_____
_____
_____

12. Place a check mark in the correct action per joint on the table below when performing PROM for the client.

| | Neck | Shoulder | Elbow | Hip | Knee |
|---|---|---|---|---|---|
| Flexion | | | | | |
| Extension | | | | | |
| Hyperextention | | | | | |
| Abduction | | | | | |
| Adduction | | | | | |
| Internal rotation | | | | | |
| External rotation | | | | | |

## Self-Assessment Questions

Circle the letter that corresponds to the best answer.

1. Clients at high risk for falls include all of the following except
   a. those with prolonged hospitalization.
   b. those taking sedatives.
   c. confused clients.
   d. those without history of physical-restraint use.

2. What is *not* a key concept to remember when positioning a client?
   a. Pressure
   b. Friction
   c. Skin color
   d. Nutrition

3. What is *not* considered a common complication of immobility?
   a. Skin breakdown
   b. Incontinence
   c. Muscle wasting
   d. Clot formation

4. Activity is important because it
   a. improves muscle tone and increases venous return.
   b. stimulates peristalsis and decreases muscle tone.
   c. is an important part of the healing process and decreases peristalsis.
   d. decreases venous return and stimulates peristalsis.

5. Of the following, the best descriptor of massage is that it
   a. cannot help rid the body of metabolic wastes.
   b. does not stimulate circulation.
   c. can open lines of communication.
   d. may detract from the therapeutic relationship.

6. M.W., a frail 80-year-old woman, is hospitalized with a stroke. She cannot move her left side. Which of the following is an indication that she should be repositioned more frequently than every two hours?
   a. Areas of redness on the right heel that resolve within 5 minutes
   b. Areas of redness on the occiput that resolve in 45 minutes
   c. When M.W. complains of constipation
   d. M.W. should only be positioned on her immobile side

7. M.W. requires a bed bath. Which of the following statements is correct when providing daily hygiene?
   a. Wash the chin and mouth area first.
   b. Cleanse the eyes from outer canthus to inner canthus.
   c. Cleanse the eyes from inner to outer canthus first.
   d. Start from the top down, so begin with her forehead.

8. The client broke his left leg in a skiing accident. The doctor ordered the client to be non–weight bearing for six-weeks. Therefore, the client needs to use crutches. Which gait should the nurse teach the client?
   a. Swing-through gait
   b. Two point gait
   c. Three-point gait
   d. Four-point gait

# Intermediate Procedures

## Key Terms

Match the following terms with their correct definitions.

___ 1. Ampule

___ 2. Catheterization

___ 3. Colostomy

___ 4. Dorsogluteal muscle

___ 5. Intramuscular injection

___ 6. Nebulizer

___ 7. Sterile technique

___ 8. Subcutaneous injection

___ 9. Vastus lateralis muscle

___ 10. Vial

a. Consists of those practices that eliminate all micro-organisms and spores from an object or area.

b. Passing a rubber or plastic tube into the bladder via the urethra.

c. An opening surgically created from the ascending, transverse, or descending colon to the abdominal wall.

d. Containers that hold a single dose of medication.

e. A small glass bottle with a rubber seal at the top.

f. Method used to administer medications into the loose connective tissues just below the dermis of the skin.

g. Method used to administer medications into the deep muscle tissue.

h. Muscle located on the anterior lateral aspect of the thigh.

i. Muscle located in the upper outer quadrant of the buttock.

j. Device that is used to aerosolize medications into a mist for delivery directly into the lungs.

## Abbreviation Review

Write the meaning or definition of the following abbreviations, acronyms, and symbols.

1. ABG _____

2. COPD _____

3. FlO2 _____

4. GI _____

5. IV _____

6. MAR _____

7. NG _____

8. OD _____

9. OR _____

10. OS _____

11. OSHA _____

12. OTC _____

13. OU _____

14. PEG _____

15. SaO2 _____

16. SMI _____

## Exercises and Activities

1. Why is open intermittent irrigation of a urinary catheter usually done?

   _____

   _____

2. What assessment findings would indicate a need for irrigation?

   _____

   _____

   _____

3. Why are heat and/or cold therapies used?

   _____

   _____

   _____

   _____

   a. What safety measures does the nurse use to protect the client during each therapy?

   Heat _____

   Cold _____

   b. What are contraindications to heat therapy?

   _____

   _____

   c. When should the nurse end the individual treatment for a client receiving heat therapy?

   _____

   _____

   d. When should the nurse end the treatment session for a client receiving cold therapy?

   _____

   _____

4. What are the seven "rights" of medication administration?

   a. _____

   b. _____

   c. _____

   d. _____

   e. _____

   f. _____

   g. _____

5. What actions should the nurse take if a client refuses a medication?

_____

_____

_____

6. What actions should the nurse take if a medication error occurs?

_____

_____

_____

7. What is the Z-track method? What medications are administered using this method?

_____

_____

_____

8. Preparations for applying a transdermal patch include:

_____

_____

_____

9. The nurse is preparing to insert an indwelling catheter before the client goes to surgery. What should the nurse say to the client about this procedure?

_____

_____

_____

   a. What position does the client need to be placed in before inserting the catheter?

   _____

   _____

   b. The nurse removes the outer wrapper and sets the catheter tray on a clean dry surface. Describe how the tray should be opened.

   _____

   _____

   c. The nurse dropped the packet of sterile betadine solution onto the floor. Describe how the nurse might handle this breach of sterile technique.

   _____

   _____

   d. If the client was female, describe how the nurse cleanses around the urinary meatus.

   _____

   _____

   e. If the client was male, describe how the nurse cleanses around the urinary meatus.

   _____

   _____

f.  What should be documented regarding the catheter insertion?

_____

_____

10. The nurse needs to administer the following medications to the client. Explain the steps of each medication:

Lanoxin 0.25 mg orally every day _____

_____

Robitussin 5 mL every 4 hours _____

_____

Fentanyl 25 mg patch every 72 hours _____

_____

11. Identify the anatomical landmarks the nurse uses to administer the following intramuscular injections:

a. Deltoid muscle  _____

b. Vastus lateralis muscle _____

c. Dorsogluteal muscle  _____

d. Ventrogluteal muscle _____

12. Explain the needle size (gauge) and angle of entry for the following types of injections.

| Site | Needle Gauge | Angle of Entry |
|------|-------------|----------------|
| Intradermal | | |
| Subcutaneous | | |
| Intramuscular | | |

13. The client has a dressing following abdominal surgery. The nurse inspects the dressing frequently. Describe what the nurse assesses the dressing for.

_____

_____

_____

a.  The wound is draining foul-smelling fluid and the physician orders a wound culture. Explain how the nurse obtains a wound culture.

_____

_____

b.  The physician decides the wound should be irrigated twice a day. What equipment should the nurse assemble for this procedure?

_____

_____

c. The nurse explains to the client the procedure of wound irrigation. How would you explain it in terms a client might understand?

_____

_____

14. The client needs to have oxygen therapy. Identify the volume of oxygen that the nurse should set each piece of equipment at.

a. Nasal cannula _____

b. Simple mask _____

c. Partial rebreather mask _____

d. Non-rebreather mask _____

e. Venturi mask _____

15. The client has a tracheostomy and requires suctioning occasionally. As the nurse prepares the equipment, what amount of suction should the wall suction unit be set at for each of the following?

For an adult: _____

For a child: _____

For an infant: _____

16. The client receives medication through a gastrostomy tube. Explain how the nurse prevents medication from clogging the tube.

_____

_____

_____

## Self-Assessment Questions

Circle the letter that corresponds to the best answer.

1. When catheterizing a client, in which hand do you hold the catheter?
   a. Right hand
   b. Left hand
   c. Either hand
   d. Dominant hand

2. What type of bladder irrigation is preferred for surgical procedures such as prostate resections?
   a. Open bladder irrigation
   b. Closed bladder irrigation
   c. Intermittent open bladder irrigation
   d. None are recommended.

3. Cold therapy can
   a. decrease blood flow to an area.
   b. increase systemic temperature.
   c. increase tissue metabolism.
   d. promote vasodilation.

4. What is the maximum amount of time a client should sit in a sitz bath?
   a. 10 minutes
   b. 15 minutes
   c. 20 minutes
   d. 25 minutes

5. When administering a douche or irrigation, the temperature should be at
   a. 90° to 95°F.
   b. 95° to 100°F.
   c. 100° to 105°F.
   d. 105° to 110°F.

# Advanced Procedures

## Key Terms

Match the following terms with their correct definitions.

___ 1. Hemophilia

___ 2. Macrodrip tubing

___ 3. Microdrip tubing

___ 4. Piggyback

___ 5. Sutures

a. Delivers 10 to 15 gtt/mL.

b. A surgical means of closing a wound, generally removed 7 to 10 days after surgery.

c. An inherited bleeding disorder.

d. Delivers 60 gtt/mL.

e. A drug that is mixed and joined to the primary IV bag.

## Abbreviation Review

Write the meaning or definition of the following abbreviations and acronyms.

1. CDC _____

2. IV _____

3. MAR _____

4. NG _____

5. NPO _____

6. ONC _____

7. OSHA _____

## Exercises and Activities

1. What are the three primary methods of obtaining blood specimens? Which is the most common?

_____

_____

_____

2. Why would a client be receiving IV fluids?

_____

_____

_____

3. What assessment signs and symptoms of an IV site would indicate infection or phlebitis?

_____

_____

_____

4. The client has a nasogastric tube. What are the reasons a client may have a nasogastric tube?

_____

_____

_____

   a. What are the two most common forms of NG tubes?

   _____

   _____

   b. Why is NG insertion a clean technique instead of a sterile one?

   _____

   _____

   c. What equipment should the nurse assemble when preparing for NG tube insertion?

   _____

   _____

   d. Describe how the nurse knows that the NG tube is correctly situated in the stomach.

   _____

   _____

5. The physician ordered an IV for the client. Why are IV fluids used instead of oral fluids?

_____

_____

_____

   a. Describe the uses for the following gauges of IV needles.
      (1) 18–19-gauge needles _____
      (2) 20–22-gauge needles _____
      (3) 22–24-gauge needles _____

   b. The nurse prepares the IV solution and the tubing but accidentally overfills the drip chamber. How should the nurse correct this?

   _____

   _____

   c. After the IV is inserted and the fluid is running freely, the client reaches to pick up a piece of paper that has fallen to the floor. The client becomes anxious when seeing blood in the IV tubing. How should the nurse respond?

   _____

   _____

   d. Describe the elements of what should be documented following IV insertion.

   _____

   _____

6. The client has a central venous catheter inserted. The nurse uses sterile technique when changing the insertion site dressing. Why is this a sterile procedure?

_____

_____

_____

7. Explain the difference between continuous and interrupted sutures.

_____

_____

_____

8. If sutures are removed too early, dehiscence may occur. Explain what dehiscence is and what the nurse should do if it occurs.

_____

_____

_____

## Self-Assessment Questions

Circle the letter that corresponds to the best answer.

1. The CDC guidelines indicate that IV tubing should be changed every
   a. 24 hours.
   b. 48 hours.
   c. 72 hours.
   d. 48–72 hours.

2. The CDC guidelines indicate that an IV site should be changed every
   a. 24 hours.
   b. 48 hours.
   c. 72 hours.
   d. 48–72 hours.

3. An order reads to administer 2 L of normal saline (NS) IV over 24 hours. The nurse has micro-drip tubing. The IV will be regulated at a rate of
   a. 42 gtt/min.
   b. 83 gtt/min.
   c. 125 gtt/min.
   d. 167 gtt/min.

4. A client is to receive an IV of 5% D/0.45 NS at 2,000 mL for 8 hours. The drip factor is 10 gtt/mL. The nurse will regulate the IV at a rate of
   a. 10 gtt/min.
   b. 21 gtt/min.
   c. 42 gtt/min.
   d. 63 gtt/min.

# Answer Key

## Chapter 1 Student Nurse Skills for Success

**Key Terms**
1. o
2. s
3. d
4. t
5. n
6. h
7. j
8. q
9. u
10. m
11. p
12. c
13. i
14. l
15. b
16. g
17. k
18. f
19. r
20. e
21. a

**Abbreviation Review**
1. blood pressure
2. computer-assisted instruction
3. National Council Licensure Examination–Practical Nursing
4. Authorization to Test
5. Unlicensed Assistive Personnel
6. The National Council of State Boards of Nursing
7. Certified Nurse Assistant

**Self-Assessment Questions**
1. c
2. d
3. c
4. a
5. b
6. c
7. d
8. b
9. b
10. d

## Chapter 2 Holistic Care

**Key Terms**
1. e
2. i
3. h
4. m
5. p
6. c
7. g
8. l
9. d
10. k
11. b
12. f
13. j
14. n
15. a
16. o

**Abbreviation Review**
1. American Holistic Nurses' Association
2. Centers for Disease Control and Prevention
3. National Institutes of Health
4. Office of Alternative Medicine

5. World Health Organization
6. National Center for Complementary and Alternative Medicine

**Self-Assessment Questions**

1. c
2. a
3. d
4. a
5. b
6. d
7. c
8. b
9. a
10. c

# Chapter 3    Nursing History, Education, and Organizations

**Key Terms**

1. b
2. k
3. h
4. a
5. l
6. e
7. g
8. d
9. j
10. i
11. c
12. f

**Abbreviation Review**

1. associate degree nurse (nursing)
2. *American Journal of Nursing*
3. American Nursing Association
4. advance practice registered nurse
5. bachelor of science in nursing
6. Certification Examination for Practical and Vocational Nurses in Long-Term Care
7. continuing education unit
8. certified in long term care
9. Council of Practical Nursing Programs
10. general education development

11. health maintenance organization
12. International Council of Nurses
13. Joint Commission on Accreditation of Healthcare Organizations
14. licensed practical nurse
15. licensed practical/vocational nurse
16. licensed vocational nurse
17. National Association of Practical Nurse Education and Service Inc.
18. National Council Licensure Examination
19. National Council of State Boards of Nursing
20. National Federation of Licensed Practical Nurses, Inc.
21. National League for Nursing
22. National League for Nursing Accrediting Commission
23. Omnibus Budget Reconciliation Act
24. registered nurse
25. Tax Equity Fiscal Responsibility Act
26. U.S. Department of Health and Human Services

**Self-Assessment Questions**

1. c
2. d
3. a
4. b
5. c
6. b
7. d
8. a
9. c
10. b

# Chapter 4   Legal and Ethical Responsibilities

**Key Terms**

1. ss
2. d
3. g
4. n
5. ww
6. aaa
7. t
8. xx
9. mm
10. vv

11. x
12. cc
13. hh
14. m
15. u
16. ee
17. bbb
18. c
19. qq
20. ddd
21. nn
22. tt
23. eee
24. w
25. h
26. v
27. hhh
28. o
29. b
30. l
31. dd
32. e
33. q
34. p
35. uu
36. gg
37. f
38. bb
39. kk
40. i
41. fff
42. y
43. jj
44. iii
45. j
46. ggg
47. ff
48. jjj
49. r
50. ii
51. z
52. s
53. aa
54. rr
55. a
56. k
57. zz
58. ll
59. oo

60. yy
61. ccc
62. pp

## Abbreviation Review

1. Americans with Disabilities Act
2. Americans Hospital Association
3. against medical advice
4. American Nurses Association
5. cardiopulmonary resuscitation
6. do not resuscitate
7. durable power of attorney for health care
8. Emergency Department
9. False Claims Act
10. Health Insurance Portability and Accountability Act
11. Health Care Integrity and Protection Data Bank
12. human immunodeficiency virus
13. International Council of Nurses
14. intramuscular
15. Joint Commission on Accreditation of Healthcare Organizations
16. licensed practical/vocational nurse
17. National Council Licensure Exam
18. National Federation of Licensed Practical Nurses
19. Protected Health Information
20. registered nurse
21. Veterans Affairs

## Self-Assessment Questions

1. c
2. d
3. b
4. a
5. b
6. d
7. a
8. b
9. a
10. b

# Chapter 5  The Health Care Delivery System

## Key Terms

1. d
2. a

3. e
4. j
5. p
6. i
7. b
8. t
9. k
10. n
11. u
12. q
13. l
14. c
15. f
16. o
17. g
18. m
19. h
20. r
21. s

## Abbreviation Review

1. Alcohol, Drug Abuse, and Mental Health Administration
2. Agency for Health Care Policy and Research
3. Agency for Health Care Research and Quality
4. acquired immunodeficiency syndrome
5. American Medical Association
6. American Nurses Association
7. advanced practice registered nurse
8. Agency for Toxic Substances and Disease Registry
9. Centers for Disease Control and Prevention
10. Children's Health Insurance Program
11. certified nurse midwife
12. community nursing organization
13. clinical nurse specialist
14. doctor of dental surgery
15. doctor of dental medicine
16. diagnosis-related group
17. exclusive provider organization
18. Food and Drug Administration
19. Health Care Financing Administration
20. health maintenance organization
21. Health Resources and Services Administration
22. Indian Health Service
23. licensed practical/vocational nurse
24. medical doctor
25. National Federation of Licensed Practical Nurses
26. National Institutes of Health
27. National League for Nursing
28. nurse practitioner
29. occupational therapist
30. physician's assistant
31. primary care provider
32. preferred provider organization
33. physical therapist
34. registered dietician
35. registered nurse
36. registered pharmacist
37. respiratory therapist
38. social worker
39. U.S. Department of Health & Human Services
40. U.S. Public Health Service
41. Veterans Administration

## Self-Assessment Questions

1. a
2. d
3. c
4. c
5. a
6. b
7. d
8. b
9. d
10. a

# Chapter 6  Arenas of Care

## Key Terms

1. d
2. i
3. g
4. a
5. f
6. c
7. h
8. d
9. e
10. j

## Abbreviation Review

1. Activities of Daily Living
2. American Health Care Association
3. Acquired Immunodeficiency Syndrome
4. Assisted Living Federation of America
5. Advanced Practice Registered Nurse
6. Commission on Accreditation of Rehabilitation Facilities
7. continuing care retirement community
8. Coronary Care Unit
9. Certification Examination for Practical and Vocational Nurses in Long-Term Care
10. community health accreditation program
11. certified in long-term care
12. computed tomography
13. extended care facility
14. Electrocardiogram
15. Emergency Department
16. Electroencephalography
17. Electromyogram
18. Health Care Finance Administration
19. health maintenance organization
20. instrumental activities of daily living
21. intermediate care facility
22. Intensive Care Unit
23. interdisciplinary health care team
24. Joint Commission on Accreditation of Healthcare Organizations
25. Magnetic Resonance Imaging
26. Omnibus Budget Reconciliation Act
27. Operating Room
28. Rural Primary Care Hospital
29. Recovery Room
30. School-Based Clinic
31. skilled nursing facility

## Self-Assessment Questions

1. c
2. a
3. d
4. b
5. c
6. c
7. a
8. b
9. d
10. c

# Chapter 7  Communication

## Key Terms

1. g
2. p
3. m
4. q
5. e
6. l
7. r
8. f
9. o
10. v
11. u
12. j
13. d
14. a
15. n
16. k
17. s
18. h
19. b
20. t
21. c
22. i

## Abbreviation Review

1. American Nurses Association
2. computerized patient record
3. human immunodeficiency virus
4. Institute of Medicine
5. words per minute

## Self-Assessment Questions

1. c
2. a
3. b
4. d
5. a
6. d
7. d
8. b
9. c
10. a

## Chapter 8  Client Teaching

### Key Terms

1. g
2. k
3. m
4. h
5. c
6. l
7. n
8. i
9. p
10. q
11. d
12. o
13. f
14. j
15. a
16. b
17. e

### Abbreviation Review

1. as evidenced by
2. Joint Commission on Accreditation of Healthcare Organizations
3. *nil per os*, Latin for "nothing by mouth"
4. related to

### Self-Assessment Questions

1. d
2. c
3. c
4. a
5. b
6. a
7. d
8. b
9. d
10. b

## Chapter 9  Nursing Process/ Documentation/ Informatics

### Key Terms

1. o
2. mm
3. u
4. n
5. rr
6. ff
7. w
8. c
9. bb
10. x
11. p
12. oo
13. d
14. i
15. gg
16. xx
17. s
18. hh
19. b
20. m
21. qq
22. nn
23. ee
24. q
25. iii
26. jj
27. h
28. ccc
29. e
30. j
31. cc
32. ww
33. aa
34. pp
35. ll
36. r
37. v
38. a
39. yy
40. t
41. vv
42. y
43. ss
44. ii
45. l
46. z
47. aaa
48. zz
49. f
50. dd
51. kk
52. g
53. uu

54. tt
55. k

## Abbreviation Review

1. as evidenced by
2. American Nurses Association
3. charting by exception
4. document, action, response
5. do not resuscitate
6. diagnosis-related group
7. hospital information system
8. Joint Commission on Accreditation of Healthcare Organizations
9. liter
10. medication administration record
11. North American Nursing Diagnosis Association
12. Nursing Interventions Classification
13. nursing information system
14. nursing minimum data set
15. Nursing Outcomes Classification
16. problem, implementation, evaluation
17. problem-oriented medical record
18. prospective payment system
19. peer review organization
20. registered nurse
21. range of motion
22. related to
23. subjective data, objective data, assessment plan
24. subjective data, objective data, assessment plan, implementation, evaluation
25. subjective data, objective data, assessment plan, implementation, evaluation, revision
26. telephone order
27. Universal Medical Language System

## Self-Assessment Questions

1. a
2. a
3. d
4. c
5. b
6. b
7. a
8. b
9. d
10. c

# Chapter 10  Life Span Development

## Key Terms

1. b
2. h
3. v
4. c
5. aa
6. i
7. x
8. n
9. d
10. y
11. o
12. r
13. j
14. bb
15. z
16. a
17. g
18. m
19. p
20. dd
21. ff
22. s
23. q
24. f
25. t
26. w
27. l
28. ee
29. u
30. cc
31. k
32. e

## Abbreviation Review

1. acquired immunodeficiency syndrome
2. breast self-exam
3. Centers for Disease Control and Prevention
4. central nervous system
5. fetal alcohol syndrome
6. phenylketonuria
7. sexually transmitted disease
8. tetanus/diphtheria
9. testicular self-exam

**Self-Assessment Questions**

1. d
2. c
3. b
4. a
5. c
6. b
7. d
8. c
9. d
10. a

# Chapter 11  Cultural Considerations

**Key Terms**

1. d
2. j
3. n
4. e
5. k
6. f
7. o
8. c
9. g
10. l
11. h
12. p
13. b
14. i
15. m
16. q
17. a

**Abbreviation Review**

1. White, Anglo-Saxon, Protestant
2. World Health Organization

**Self-Assessment Questions**

1. c
2. a
3. d
4. b
5. b
6. d
7. b
8. d
9. c
10. a

# Chapter 12  Stress, Adaptation, and Anxiety

**Key Terms**

1. b
2. f
3. k
4. o
5. a
6. p
7. r
8. c
9. e
10. x
11. j
12. l
13. q
14. u
15. s
16. w
17. g
18. m
19. t
20. v
21. i
22. d
23. n
24. h

**Abbreviation Review**

1. cerebral vascular accident
2. general adaptation syndrome
3. local adaptation syndrome
4. North American Nursing Diagnosis Association

**Self-Assessment Questions**

1. a
2. c
3. a
4. b
5. d
6. b
7. b
8. a
9. c
10. d

## Chapter 13  End-of-Life Care

### Key Terms

1. cc
2. i
3. m
4. v
5. f
6. p
7. a
8. j
9. w
10. q
11. b
12. bb
13. aa
14. r
15. x
16. d
17. k
18. u
19. e
20. l
21. z
22. n
23. g
24. s
25. o
26. h
27. y
28. c
29. t

### Abbreviation Review

1. American Nurses Association
2. do not resuscitate
3. health maintenance organization
4. intramuscular
5. morphine sulfate
6. North American Nursing Diagnosis Association
7. Omnibus Budget Reconciliation Act
8. Patient Self-Determination Act
9. post-traumatic stress disorder
10. sudden infant death syndrome
11. tuberculosis

### Self-Assessment Questions

1. c
2. a
3. b
4. d
5. c
6. c
7. a
8. d
9. c
10. b

## Chapter 14  Wellness Concepts

### Key Terms

1. g
2. c
3. d
4. f
5. a
6. e
7. b

### Abbreviation Review

1. acquired immunodeficiency syndrome
2. Body Mass Index
3. Centers for Disease Control and Prevention
4. electrocardiogram
5. electrocardiogram
6. hemoglobin
7. human immunodeficiency virus
8. low density lipoprotein
9. papanicolau test
10. Public Health Service
11. sun protection factor
12. United States Department of Health and Human Services
13. World Health Organization

### Self-Assessment Questions

1. c
2. b
3. a
4. b
5. c
6. b
7. d
8. d
9. c
10. d

## Chapter 15  Self-Concept

**Key Terms**
1. a
2. e
3. i
4. k
5. b
6. a
7. h
8. g
9. c
10. f
11. j

**Abbreviation Review**
1. North American Nursing Diagnosis Association

**Self-Assessment Questions**
1. b
2. a
3. a
4. c
5. d

## Chapter 16  Spirituality

**Key Terms**
1. h
2. e
3. c
4. b
5. g
6. d
7. i
8. a
9. f

**Abbreviation Review**
1. American Nurses Association
2. North American Nursing Diagnosis Association

**Self-Assessment Questions**
1. b
2. b
3. d
4. b
5. c

## Chapter 17  Complementary/Alternative Therapies

**Key Terms**
1. f
2. m
3. z
4. d
5. w
6. l
7. g
8. n
9. k
10. a
11. x
12. r
13. y
14. h
15. b
16. j
17. i
18. o
19. t
20. e
21. p
22. c
23. v
24. q
25. s
26. u

**Abbreviation Review**
1. Animal-Assisted therapy
2. Complementary/alternative
3. Food and Drug Administration
4. National Center for Complementary and Alternative Medicine
5. National Institutes of Health
6. progressive muscle relaxation
7. psychoneuroimmunoendocrinology

**Self-Assessment Questions**
1. a
2. d
3. a
4. b
5. c
6. c

7. b
8. a
9. c
10. c

# Chapter 18 Basic Nutrition

**Key Terms**

1. h
2. a
3. m
4. gg
5. x
6. d
7. hh
8. mm
9. oo
10. cc
11. e
12. n
13. r
14. ee
15. jj
16. pp
17. vv
18. uu
19. s
20. tt
21. aa
22. ll
23. b
24. t
25. l
26. nn
27. qq
28. v
29. bb
30. ff
31. kk
32. xx
33. c
34. rr
35. zz
36. ii
37. i
38. w
39. aaa
40. k
41. ww
42. q
43. bbb
44. o
45. y
46. dd
47. ss
48. f
49. u
50. ccc
51. z
52. yy
53. g
54. p
55. ddd
56. j

**Abbreviation Review**

1. adequate intake
2. body mass index
3. carbohydrate (carbon, hydrogen, oxygen)
4. protein (carbon, hydrogen, oxygen, nitrogen)
5. chloride
6. central nervous system
7. deciliter
8. deoxyribonucleic acid
9. dietary reference intake
10. estimated average requirement
11. extracellular fluid
12. Food and Drug Administration
13. Iron
14. foot
15. gram
16. gastrointestinal
17. intake and output
18. intracellular fluid
19. inch
20. Potassium
21. kilocalorie
22. kilogram
23. pound
24. Magnesium
25. milligram
26. milliliter
27. Sodium
28. nasogastric
29. Nutrition, Labeling, and Education Act
30. *nil per os*, Latin for "nothing by mouth"
31. ounce

32. Phosphorus
33. red blood cell
34. recommended dietary allowances
35. ribonucleic acid
36. Sulfur
37. tube feeding
38. total parental nutrition
39. upper intake level
40. U.S. Department of Agriculture
41. white blood cell
42. Zinc

**Self-Assessment Questions**
1. a
2. d
3. b
4. a
5. c
6. d
7. b
8. d
9. c
10. a

# Chapter 19  Rest and Sleep

**Key Terms**
1. n
2. d
3. m
4. g
5. l
6. a
7. h
8. i
9. b
10. j
11. f
12. k
13. c
14. e
15. p
16. q
17. r
18. o

**Abbreviation Review**
1. continuous positive airway pressure
2. electroencephalograph

3. North American Nursing Diagnosis
4. non-rapid eye movement
5. National Sleep Foundation
6. Nocturnal Sleep-Related Eating Disorder
7. periodic limb movement in sleep
8. premenstrual syndrome
9. rapid eye movement
10. restless leg syndrome

**Self Assessment Questions**
1. c
2. d
3. b
4. a
5. d
6. b
7. b
8. d
9. c
10. a

# Chapter 20  Safety/Hygiene

**Key Terms**
1. d
2. j
3. c
4. e
5. h
6. b
7. k
8. n
9. g
10. a
11. l
12. i
13. f
14. m

**Abbreviation Review**
1. activities of daily living
2. Centers for Disease Control and Prevention
3. coronary heart disease
4. Centers for Medicare and Medicaid Services
5. cardiopulmonary resuscitation
6. Food and Drug Administration
7. Glasgow Coma Scale

8. high density lipoprotein
9. identification
10. Joint of Accreditation of Healthcare Organizations
11. material safety data sheet
12. North American Nursing Diagnosis Association
13. Omnibus Budget Reconciliation Act
14. Occupational Safety and Health Administration
15. patient-controlled analgesia

**Self-Assessment Questions**
1. a
2. d
3. c
4. d
5. b
6. c
7. d
8. b
9. a
10. c

# Chapter 21 Infection Control/ Asepsis

**Key Terms**
1. d
2. oo
3. x
4. ii
5. tt
6. rr
7. z
8. aaa
9. qq
10. k
11. pp
12. q
13. hh
14. w
15. u
16. r
17. y
18. e
19. ff
20. ss
21. zz
22. jj
23. xx
24. c
25. j
26. v
27. p
28. bbb
29. aa
30. kk
31. gg
32. ccc
33. f
34. mm
35. vv
36. cc
37. b
38. ll
39. l
40. s
41. ww
42. yy
43. i
44. nn
45. dd
46. o
47. ee
48. g
49. t
50. uu
51. m
52. bb
53. a
54. h
55. n

**Abbreviation Review**
1. acquired immunodeficiency syndrome
2. Association for Professionals in Infection Control and Epidemiology
3. Centers for Disease Control and Prevention
4. deoxyribonucleic acid
5. Environmental Protection Agency
6. erythrocyte sedimentation rate
7. hepatitis B virus
8. hepatitis C virus
9. human immunodeficiency virus
10. North American Nursing Disgnosis Association

11. operating room
12. Occupational Safety and Health Administration
13. potential hydrogen
14. ribonucleic acid
15. tuberculosis
16. white blood cell, white blood count

**Self-Assessment Questions**
1. d
2. b
3. c
4. a
5. d
6. a
7. d
8. c
9. b
10. a

# Chapter 22  Standard Precautions and Isolation

**Key Terms**

1. c
2. i
3. k
4. d
5. f
6. h
7. l
8. g
9. a
10. b
11. j
12. e

**Abbreviation Review**
1. acquired immunodeficiency syndrome
2. body substance isolation
3. Centers for Disease Control and Prevention
4. Department of Health and Human Services
5. hepatitis B virus

6. Hospital Infection Control Practices Advisory Committee
7. human immunodeficiency virus
8. multidrug-resistant
9. Occupational Safety and Health Administration
10. tuberculosis

**Self-Assessment Questions**
1. b
2. c
3. d
4. a
5. b
6. c
7. b
8. a
9. c
10. d

# Chapter 23  Bioterrorism

**Key Terms**
1. c
2. m
3. l
4. g
5. k
6. d
7. i
8. j
9. n
10. f
11. e
12. h
13. a
14. b
15. o

**Abbreviation Review**
1. Centers for Disease Control and Prevention
2. Chemical, Biological, Radiological/ Nuclear, and Explosive Enhanced Response Force Package
3. Expeditionary Medical Support
4. Emergency operations plan
5. Federal Emergency Management Agency

6. potassium iodide
7. Strategic National Stockpile
8. Vendor-managed inventory
9. Nerve agents

### Self-Assessment Questions
1. a
2. b
3. b
4. a
5. a

## Chapter 24  Fluid, Electrolyte, and Acid-Base Balance

### Key Terms
1. oo
2. t
3. cc
4. pp
5. e
6. dd
7. s
8. f
9. bb
10. qq
11. g
12. rr
13. h
14. r
15. u
16. ee
17. v
18. tt
19. kk
20. gg
21. n
22. m
23. b
24. ss
25. ff
26. a
27. i
28. p
29. w
30. ll
31. o
32. uu
33. c
34. x
35. aa
36. d
37. mm
38. q
39. z
40. hh
41. j
42. ii
43. nn
44. vv
45. y
46. k
47. jj
48. l

### Fill in the Blank
1. anion
2. cation
3. ion
4. atom

### Abbreviation Review

1. arterial blood gases
2. antidiuretic hormone
3. adenosine triphosphatase
4. blood pressure
5. blood urea nitrogen
6. calcium ion
7. complete blood count
8. chloride ion
9. carbon dioxide ion
10. carboxyl group
11. central nervous system
12. dextrose 5% in water
13. deciliter
14. extracellular fluid
15. gastrointestinal
16. hydrogen ion
17. carbonic acid
18. water
19. hydrochloric acid
20. bicarbonate ion
21. hematocrit
22. hemoglobin
23. intake and output

24. intracellular fluid
25. intravenous
26. potassium ion
27. potassium chloride
28. kilogram
29. liter
30. pound
31. milliequivalent
32. milligram
33. magnesium ion
34. milliliter
35. millimeters of mercury
36. Milk of Magnesia
37. milliosmoles/kilogram
38. sodium ion
39. sodium chloride
40. sodium dihydrogen phosphate
41. sodium bicarbonate
42. sodium monohydrogen phosphate
43. sodium hydroxide
44. amino group
45. nothing by mouth
46. oxygen
47. hydroxyl
48. partial pressure of carbon dioxide
49. potential hydrogen
50. partial pressure of oxygen
51. phosphate ion
52. oxygen saturation
53. total parenteral nutrition
54. temperature, pulse, respirations
55. weight

## Self-Assessment Questions

1. d
2. a
3. b
4. a
5. c
6. a
7. b
8. b
9. c
10. d

# Chapter 25  Medication Administration and IV Therapy

## Key Terms

1. n
2. v
3. g
4. ee
5. u
6. o
7. kk
8. a
9. ff
10. i
11. jj
12. t
13. ii
14. pp
15. oo
16. gg
17. bb
18. b
19. s
20. j
21. c
22. f
23. w
24. dd
25. ll
26. mm
27. p
28. e
29. x
30. cc
31. y
32. m
33. d
34. z
35. l
36. q
37. h
38. aa
39. nn
40. hh
41. k
42. r

**Fill in the Blank**
1. *United States Pharmacopia/National Formulary*
2. generic
3. parenteral route
4. absorption

**Abbreviation Review**
1. acquired immunodeficiency syndrome
2. body surface area
3. cup
4. cubic centimeter
5. centimeter
6. central venous catheter
7. dextrose 5% in water
8. Drug Enforcement Agency
9. dram, or ʒ
10. Food and Drug Administration
11. fluid
12. gram
13. gastrointestinal
14. grain
15. drops
16. intradermal
17. intramuscular
18. intravenous
19. intravenous piggyback
20. kilogram
21. keep vein open
22. liter
23. pound
24. ♏
25. medication administration record
26. microgram, or μg
27. milligram
28. minute
29. milliliter
30. *National Formulary*
31. nasogastric
32. nothing by mouth
33. nitroglycerin
34. ounce or ʒ?
35. *per os*, Latin for "by mouth"
36. Latin for "as needed"
37. pint
38. prothrombin time
39. partial thromboplastin time
40. everyday
41. quart

42. red blood cell, red blood count
43. subcutaneous
44. teaspoon
45. tablespoon
46. *United States Pharmacopeia*
47. vascular access device

**Self-Assessment Questions**
1. b
2. c
3. a
4. b
5. a
6. b
7. c
8. d
9. b
10. c

# Chapter 26  Assessment

**Key Terms**
1. i
2. u
3. l
4. a
5. m
6. v
7. dd
8. s
9. j
10. d
11. cc
12. t
13. k
14. ff
15. z
16. w
17. ee
18. b
19. n
20. f
21. bb
22. o
23. e
24. p
25. r
26. y
27. q

28. h
29. c
30. x
31. g
32. aa

**Abbreviation Review**

1. blood pressure
2. centimeter
3. left lower quadrant
4. level of consciousness
5. left upper quadrant
6. pulse
7. pupils equal, round, reactive to light and accommodation
8. respiration
9. right lower quadrant
10. review of systems
11. right upper quadrant
12. temperature

**Self-Assessment Questions**

1. b
2. c
3. d
4. a
5. c
6. b
7. d
8. c
9. a
10. b

# Chapter 27  Pain Management

**Key Terms**

1. hh
2. a
3. g
4. bb
5. aa
6. ii
7. rr
8. kk
9. b
10. gg
11. jj

12. h
13. y
14. j
15. c
16. z
17. i
18. ll
19. k
20. cc
21. t
22. f
23. o
24. mm
25. p
26. dd
27. n
28. e
29. u
30. ff
31. v
32. d
33. m
34. w
35. l
36. x
37. oo
38. qq
39. ee
40. s
41. r
42. q
43. nn
44. pp

**Abbreviation Review**

1. American Pain Society
2. Agency for Health Care Policy and Research
3. around the clock
4. eutectic (cream) mixture of local anesthetics
5. International Association for the Study of Pain
6. magnetic resonance imaging
7. *nil per os*, Latin for "nothing by mouth"
8. nonsteroidal anti-inflammatory drug
9. patient-controlled analgesic
10. *pro re nata*, Latin for "as required"

11. tetracaine, adrenaline, cocaine
12. transcutaneous electrical nerve stimulation
13. temporomandibular joint
14. Visual Analog Scale
15. World Health Organization

**Self-Assessment Questions**
1. a
2. b
3. b
4. c
5. d
6. b
7. a
8. c
9. d
10. a

# Chapter 28  Diagnostic Tests

**Key Terms**
1. l
2. x
3. k
4. tt
5. kk
6. a
7. m
8. n
9. vv
10. jj
11. y
12. ss
13. d
14. o
15. e
16. ff
17. i
18. w
19. ll
20. qq
21. j
22. mm
23. uu
24. oo
25. b
26. ii
27. c
28. aa
29. p
30. rr
31. q
32. aaa
33. z
34. gg
35. ee
36. h
37. u
38. dd
39. v
40. ww
41. hh
42. g
43. t
44. cc
45. xx
46. zz
47. s
48. nn
49. yy
50. f
51. bb
52. pp
53. r

**Abbreviation Review**
1. arterial blood gas
2. culture and sensitivity
3. cerebrospinal fluid
4. computed tomography
5. electrocardiogram
6. electroencephalogram
7. intravenous pyelogram
8. partial pressure of carbon dioxide
9. partial pressure of oxygen
10. red blood cell, red blood count
11. white blood cell, white blood count

**Self-Assessment Questions**
1. c
2. a
3. b
4. d
5. c
6. d
7. b
8. b

9. d
10. c

## Chapter 29  Basic Procedures

**Key Terms**
1. e
2. m
3. k
4. c
5. d
6. a
7. f
8. b
9. i
10. j
11. h
12. g
13. l

**Abbreviation Review**
1. Airway, breathing, circulation, defibrillation
2. Automated External Defibrillator
3. Centers for Disease Control and Prevention
4. Cardiopulmonary resuscitation
5. Emergency Medical System
6. Intake and Output
7. Point of maximal impulse
8. Passive range of motion
9. Range of motion
10. Vancomycin-resistant enterococci

**Self-Assessment Questions**
1. d
2. d
3. b
4. a
5. c
6. b
7. c
8. a

## Chapter 30  Intermediate Procedures

**Key Terms**
1. d
2. b
3. c
4. i
5. g
6. j
7. a
8. f
9. h
10. e

**Abbreviation Review**
1. Arterial blood gas
2. Chronic obstructive pulmonary disease
3. Fraction of inspired oxygen
4. Gastrointestinal
5. Intravenous
6. Medication administration record
7. Nasogastric
8. Right eye
9. Operating room
10. Left eye
11. Occupational Safety and Health Administration
12. Over-the-counter
13. Both eyes
14. Percutaneous endoscopic gastrostomy
15. Arterial blood oxygen saturation
16. Sustained maximum inspiration

**Self -Assessment Questions**
1. d
2. b
3. a
4. c
5. d

## Chapter 31  Advanced Procedures

**Key Terms**
1. c
2. a
3. d
4. e
5. b

**Abbreviation Review**
1. Centers for Disease Control and Prevention
2. Intravenous
3. Medication administration record
4. Nasogastric
5. Nothing by mouth
6. Over-the-needle catheter
7. Occupational Safety and Health Administration

**Self-Assessment Questions**
1. b
2. d
3. b
4. c